Beauty

Confidential

By Nadine Haobsh

BEAUTY CONFIDENTIAL

Beauty

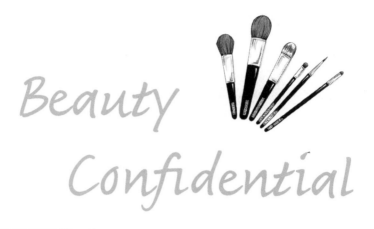

Confidential

The no preaching, no lies, advice-you'll-actually-use guide to looking your best

Nadine Haobsh

AVON

An Imprint of HarperCollins*Publishers*

The views expressed herein are the author's own; the publisher and the author expressly disclaim liability for any damages resulting from the application of the information in this book.

Index of Products appears on pages 275–285.

HarperCollins books may be purchased for educational, business, or sales promotional use. For information please write: Special Markets Department, HarperCollins Publishers, 10 East 53rd Street, New York, NY 10022.

FIRST EDITION

Designed by Elizabeth Glover
Illustrations by Kara Strubel

Library of Congress Cataloging-in-Publication Data

Haobsh, Nadine.
    Beauty confidential : the no preaching, no lies, advice-you'll-actually-use guide to looking your best / Nadine Haobsh. — 1st ed.
        p. cm.
Includes bibliographical references and index.
ISBN: 978-0-06-112863-9
ISBN–10: 0-06-112863-5
1. Beauty, Personal.   2. Cosmetics.   I. Title.

RA778.H233   2007
646.7'042—dc22   2007014800

07   08   09   10   11   DT/RRD   10   9   8   7   6   5   4   3   2

Acknowledgments

Billions of thanks to my family—Nancy, Fred, and Pierre—for letting me gallivant all over the world from an exceedingly young age, rewarding me as a child with books, having confidence in my choices, providing financial support after my blog *scandale*, and never once making me doubt myself. I love you.

To everybody at HarperCollins and William Morris, a big thanks, especially to my brilliant editor, Carrie Feron, and my patient, beyond helpful agent, Dorian Karchmar. I cannot sing your praises enough. To Jesse Fuller, I could spend the next forty-five pages thanking you for all that you've done, but for now I'll say thanks for pulling it all together on a dime and being there for me 24/7 and leave it at that. Steven Beer, thank you so much for your guidance and friendship through it all. Jonathan Pecarsky, your early support and enthusiasm was so appreciated. Special thanks to Sophie Dawson, without whom I possibly may have had a nervous breakdown and been forced to flee the country until my deadline had passed. You were a godsend.

Sarah Gilmour, Courtney Sauve, Jamie Stone, Kaiti Hryb and Lauren Williams—I thank you from the bottom of my heart.

To Amy Gibson, Michi Gracida and Dara Smith, who read, re-read, listened patiently as I babbled about mascara, allowed me to attack them at whim with hairdryers, and provided much-needed moral support, thank you. I will keep you stocked with lip gloss for the rest of your lives.

Thanks to my experts and beauty gurus: Ted Gibson, Kristen Vincelli, Kathy Galotti, Mark Garrison, Nick Barose, Shalini Vadhera, Dr. Kenneth Beer, Dr. Dennis Gross, Oribe, Edward Tricomi, Carol Shaw, Louise Galvin, Eliut Rivera, and Elke Von Freudenberg.

Patricia Reynoso, I'm sorry for letting you down. You were, and remain, an inspiration.

To "the Boss," who changed my life forever: thank you. It means more than you could possibly know.

And to all the rest who had a hand—whether you realized it or not!—I couldn't have done it without you: Jessica Coen, Jessica Cutler, Adrienne Elker, Emily Fink, Susanna Fogel, Jean Godfrey-June, Carlos Gracida, Julio, Memo and Mimi Gracida, Deenie Hartzog, David Hauslaib, Perez Hilton, Steve Hofstetter, Ron Hogan, Brandon Holley, Allison Intondi, Faran Krentcil, Andrew Krucoff, Melissa Ladsky, Michael Malice, Katherine McKenney, Erica Metzger, Robyn Meyer, Raakhee Mirchandani, Brandusa Niro, Jesse Oxfeld, Brooke Parkhurst, Camille

Payne, Wendy Powers, Patricia Reynoso, Holly Siegel, Kristin Sikorski, Rachel Sklar, Katherine Snedden, Frank Vivolo, Jordan Warren, Tessa Woodward, and every publicist who has me on their mailing list. Without you, the industry would grind to a halt. No face cream? No purses? You are the unsung heroes.

Contents

Beauty
Confidential

Introduction

For five years, I worked as a beauty editor in New York City, swinging my way from magazine to magazine and quickly working my way up the masthead. I was on track to becoming a beauty director—one of the younger ones in the industry, if things kept course. Then I started writing a blog called "Jolie in NYC." And then all hell broke loose.

My blog was a poor-man's version of the popular gossip sites that were sprouting like kudzu, with regurgitated celebrity news that I posted and added my own hi-*larious* two cents on. I even enjoyed a brief side foray into the public service sector, cobbling together a side blog called "Nick and Jessica Breakup Watch," which included proof of their imminent demise. (Hey, I *was* right in the end.) After taking a particularly lavish press trip to Arizona, however, I briefly tabled the celebrity content and wrote instead about our journey, marveling at how beauty editors were treated to such perks as private jets, designer handbags, and massages. The blog was anonymous (mistake one) and included commentary on my industry and the often tenuous dynamics between editors and publicists (mistake two). I started getting coverage in blogs like Gawker, Jossip, and Mediabistro, was swiftly outed by the *New York Post*, and had a plum offer at *Seventeen* magazine rescinded . . . the day after I left my position at *Ladies' Home Journal.* (Worst . . . day . . . of . . . my . . . life.)

Except, in retrospect, it wasn't. I learned that flexibility and hard work are not mutually exclusive and decided on a whim to go for broke, trying to make a career out of this craaazy blogging thing. (Cue violins.) Every second I could, I posted, noting favorite products, great tips gleaned from industry experts, celebrity beauty trends, and, most importantly, answering beauty questions from readers. In the flurry of Q&A's, I realized that there's a serious lack of *honesty* in today's beauty information: we're sick of being lectured, talked down to, advertised at, and just generally misled.

The questions are endless. When every dermatologist in America is touting an astronomically pricey skin-care line, does that mean you're ruining your complexion if you only have money for the drugstore stuff? Why do all the magazines champion that product you spent two hundred dollars on, when it did absolutely *nothing* for you? Why does it feel like you read the same beauty article every single month, in every single magazine? Isn't it a strange coincidence that the product you're reading about on page 53 is advertised on page 55? And why is it so hard to grasp that the label "combination skin" helps nobody? (Fine, you're dry here, you're oily there, but all of the "right" products either make you flake or break out!)

I set out to create a beauty book for *you*—the girl who loves makeup, hair, perfume, and skin care, but wants to find what works for her without blindly following trends or swallowing corporate-placement rubbish. There are millions of beauty books on the shelves by experts, crammed with step-by-step instructions on how to painstakingly create the look that will make you appear as if you've just stepped from the pages of your favorite magazine. While that's fabulous, if you have time to read a complicated manual the size of a World War Two textbook and then spend hours aping the looks inside . . . most of us don't! We want fast, accurate, and *real*, and we want it from somebody who's been there in the beauty trenches with us. Let's be honest: I'm not a makeup artist, I'm not a hairstylist, and I've singed my hair, poked out my eyes, and turned myself orange more times than I'd like to count! But I *have* been surrounded by beauty information 24/7 for several years, and armed with enough knowledge to make over an entire village of frizzy-haired, oily t-zoned, crying-out-in-need-of-highlights women, I hereby pass it all along to you.

Thanks for reading, and stay beautiful!

One

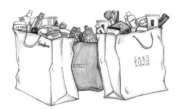

Getting Started

What beauty editors know that you don't

Imagine a life where highlights and haircuts with the world's top experts are free, where there is an endless supply of Crème de la Mer, where you leave work at 2 P.M. to get a massage or pedicure and your boss cheerfully tells you to have fun. (Are you still with me?) Now, imagine you get *paid* to live this life. Welcome to the world of a beauty editor.

Each month, magazines bring you advice on which eye shadow shades are hot, what the most flattering haircut is for your face shape, and which self-tanners work for pale skin. But have you ever wondered how beauty editors know all this? (For me, it's because I was born knowing everything there is to know about beauty. *Obviously.*) In reality, it's because beauty experts have free products and procedures hurled at them. It may not seem fair—why do they get endless supplies of Chanel lip gloss, and all you get at work is an endless supply of paperclips? —but expertise is the name of the game. Without batting an eyelash, a beauty editor can tell you definitively what the best cleanser is, how to get away with not washing your hair for four days, what on earth a peptide is, why the jasmine in perfumes is picked at night, and the difference between alpha and beta hydroxy acid. The advice you see in magazines each month is just a fraction of the actual knowledge they possess.

I'm here to share it with you.

I wasn't always beauty-savvy. A childhood spent climbing avocado trees and shunning Barbies in favor of books does not necessarily a future beauty editor make. But in college, while pursuing a career as a writer, I found myself at a magazine as a beauty intern. The first time I walked into the magical thing known as a beauty closet, I almost fainted. Much like that episode of *Sex and the City* where Carrie goes to *Vogue* and has a heart attack over the fabulosity of the fashion closet, I was shocked to see that the room (Yes! An entire room!) was stuffed to the

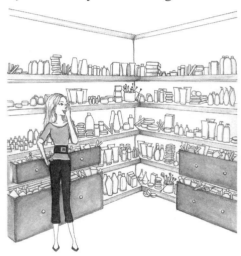

brim with every product known to man. Better yet, it was ours for the sampling. After all, how are you going to be a beauty expert if you don't try all the products?

There are thousands of beauty products in this world (Hundreds of thousands! Millions!), and your average girl can't be expected to try them all. So, we tireless beauty editors do the work for you, dutifully slapping on face cream, testing hair straighteners, and staring intently at nearly identical shades of lip gloss, trying to figure out which is better for olive complexions and which for fairer skin tones.

See? And you thought it was all fun and games. Beauty is *very serious.*

Actually, I'm kidding. Most people take beauty way too seriously, and it simply doesn't need to be that way. Beauty should be fun! It should make you feel better about yourself and accentuate what you've been blessed with (and gracefully and discreetly hide what you're less than pleased with). All that nonsense about "redheads can't wear red lipstick" and "don't match your manicure to your pedicure" and "young women shouldn't wear foundation" and "never play up your eyes and lips at the same time" is just that—nonsense. It's all about finding what works for *you.* If you're in your teens or twenties and your skin is slightly blotchy and tinted moisturizer simply doesn't give you enough coverage, I say wear foundation until the cows come home! The trick is simply finding the *right* foundation that doesn't make you feel like you have on a mask.

It's not rocket science, people. Sure, beauty is serious in that it's terribly important for your self-esteem. Like it or not, we do live in an image-conscious society, and why not put your best face forward? But, after all, at the end of the day, it *is* only makeup. Lighten up, don't be afraid to experiment and make mistakes, and have fun with it!

And when your friends ask you how you know all about night-blooming jasmine and peptides, well, you can just smile and say that you were born a beauty genius.

∽ First Things First

Beauty editors are very stern about certain things. Now, I don't necessarily live my life according to all of the Stepford-ish maxims, but rather take them as loose guidelines. After all, there are exceptions to *every* rule . . .

The Beauty Editor Commandments

1. Never wash your hair two days in a row.

2. Always wear SPF 30 sunscreen, come rain or shine, winter or summer.

3. Wash your face every night before bed . . . even when drunk . . . even when tired.

4. French manicures are not an option.

5. Everybody looks better with a hint of bronzer or self-tanner.

6. Avoid frowning—just like your mom said, your face will stick that way.

7. Don't smoke—it causes wrinkles, sallow, uneven skin, and yellow teeth. (Oh, yeah, and that whole cancer thing, too.)

8. Introduce acids into your daily routine—glycolic, salicylic, retinoic, whatever. Your skin will thank you.

9. Antioxidants are your best friend. Eat them, drink them, wear them, love them.

10. Smile. When you carry yourself beautiful, you <u>are</u> beautiful.

∾ But, Hey, They're Only People, Too

There are some silly things that beauty editors are unnecessarily sticklers about, such as nail polish shades (never wear red on your nails!) and shampooing (see above!). While this is good advice, say, if you're a banker—who's going to take you seriously with fire-engine-red claws?—one size does not fit all. My best friend has oily, limp hair, and no amount of volumizer or hair powder is going to allow her to skip a day between washes as is normally recommended. As for the "no red nails" maxim, well—that's just foolish. (A life without red nail polish is no life at all.) Become as beauty informed as you can, and take everything you read (hey, even this) with a grain of salt. Everyone is unique and reacts to different products and tips in different ways. If we were all completely the same, where would the fun be in that? Variety is the spice of life, after all.

∾ Becoming a Beauty "Expert": Or, The Road to Beauty Enlightenment

As a beauty editor, you have the keys to the city, metaphorically speaking. Just received a story assignment on perfumes? Call Chanel, Hermès, Dior, Guerlain, and Givenchy, and within three hours, you'll have a sampling waiting in your office of the most exclusive fragrances known to man. Have a weakness for products by Bobbi Brown, Clarins, Stila, or the Body Shop? Simply shoot the publicist an email explaining that you'd like to try out the new face cream, or that you've just run out of your favorite eyeliner. Forgot to buy mom a birthday present? Rummage through the beauty closet until you've unearthed a Diptyque candle in Baies, a jar of Crème de la Mer, and the entire Calvin Klein Eternity Moment ancillary line.

When I first learned that, as an assistant, I was allowed—nay! expected!—not only to call in products but to actually *try them out*, I was stunned. You mean . . . publicists would send me beauty products . . . *for free*? It boggled the mind. Still more shocking was the revelation that all spa and salon services—we're talking haircuts, highlights, blowouts, glazes, massages, manicures, and pedicures—were on the house. Why? Well, after all, how can you be expected to write about it if you haven't tried it?

I went nuts. I hit every salon in town. I took my already blond hair blonder. (Much satisfaction ensued when one colorist had to stop mid-highlight to "take a call from Nicole." As in Kidman.) I made it red. I made it black. I cut it all off. I had extensions put in. I got bangs. Then I went back to the exact same color and hairstyle I'd started off with when I got into the industry, satisfied that I had, quite literally, done it all. With the salon options exhausted, I dipped into spa services—a chocolate pedicure here, a paraffin wax manicure there, and all of the massages, professional self-tanning, waxing and lasering my little body could stand. At one point, with my long, blond, Paris Hilton–style extensions, fake tan, hairless body, "color-enhancing" blue contact lenses and glossy nails, I looked like a Barbie doll come to life. I thought I was beyond glamorous. My friends thought I had gone off the deep end.

The problem was that beauty was consuming me. In the quest to become as stereotypically pretty as possible, I was completely erasing *me*. For every gorgeous "perfect" celebrity like Halle Berry, Elizabeth Taylor, Elle MacPherson, or Charlize Theron, there have been an equal number of "imperfect" goddesses that have captivated our imaginations. Can you imagine Gisele Bundchen with a ski-jump nose? Keira Knightley with a D cup? Beyoncé Knowles with a nonexistent booty? Barbara Streisand without her famous profile? Lucy Liu with "Western" eyes? Lauren Hutton without that sexy gap? I don't want to. Those so-called flaws have inspired generations of girls with similar features to look in the mirror and say, "You know what? I *am* pretty—just the way I am."

Even I don't wake up looking like Cindy Crawford.

Cindy Crawford

However, while I champion easy, natural, accessible beauty, I don't believe in being judgmental about it. It's not about scoffing at other's choices, saying, "Well, *I* would never do that" and feeling superior as a result. If you have healthy self-esteem, but simply feel that you'd look better with, say, a nose job, or breast implants, or Botox injections—to each her own. To quote a famous Sheryl Crow song, "If it makes you happy, it can't be that bad." Life is just too short to spend obsessing about various imperfections. I say either learn to love 'em, or change them and move on. Simple as that.

(Important point: Just because I'm now all wannabe-zen about beauty doesn't mean I'm not still a product junkie. The excitement over Chanel perfume never fades, no matter *what* you look like.)

∾ "MUST" LIST: The Products in Every Beauty Editor's Cabinet

Some beauty editors are drugstore gals, others love department store goodies, still more are verifiable snobs, only using products that cost more than the GDP of a small country. Whatever each gal's preferences, however, a few products exist that are just *so* effective, you're guaranteed to find them in every single beauty editor's cabinet.

NARS blush in Orgasm: A peachy-rose, universally beloved, makes-every-woman-look-sexy-no-matter-what-her-complexion, no-other-product-can-even-come-close, rock-star blush. The name pretty much says it all—it gives you the kind of subtle, naughty flush that only comes from . . . well . . . you know.

Terax Original Crema: Is there a better intensive conditioner in the world? If so, I have yet to find it. Crema works miracles on dry, overprocessed hair, turning it from straw into silk. Bonus points because it's Italian and has an innate glamor quotient. (Maybe it shouldn't matter, but, c'mon—it *so* does.)

Essie Mademoiselle and OPI I'm Not Really a Waitress nail polish: With these two nail polish shades in your kit, you're pretty much set for life. Mademoiselle is the ideal pale pink—not too white, not too rose—that goes everywhere and immediately makes nails look Rich Bitch chic; I'm Not Really a Waitress fulfils the elusive, eternal quest for the perfect red.

Mario Badescu Drying Potion: When it's Thursday night, you have the biggest date of your life on Friday, and a zit the size of Mount Vesuvius has suddenly erupted, look no further than this tiny bottle of Pepto Bismol–pink pimple destroyer. Within one evening, the blemish will be considerably reduced; if you're lucky enough to have two nights to spare, it'll be nearly gone. (And three nights? Zit? What zit?)

Shu Uemura Eyelash Curler: Okay, so it kind of looks like a mechanical torture device. Don't let that scare you. Use before applying mascara and your eyelashes will be twice as defined, as if by magic. It's the best thing this side of false lashes.

Bumble and bumble Does It All Styling Spray: Whether your hair is curly or straight, frizzy or limp, thick or thin, this styling and setting spray lives up to its name. It doubles as a medium-hold hairspray, keeping tresses in place without any gross, beauty-pageant–like stiffness, but easily brushes out and works fabulously with heat-styling tools.

Cetaphil Face Wash: Dermatologists swear by it for a reason—it's gentle enough for even the most sensitive, dry, or trouble-prone skin. When the mere thought of washing your face is enough to make your skin inflamed, this is your product. Beloved whether you're sixteen or sixty.

Kiehl's Lip Balm # 1: Combats chapped lips like nobody's business, lasts for hours, and comes in both a pot and a tube version. Plus, it's unisex and scent-free, so the man in your life won't whine that you taste like a mango-pomegranate-kiwi (and then will probably steal it for himself).

Lancôme Definicils: While other mascaras might get more press, this remains the gold standard, lengthening, defining, and just generally tricking-out even the wimpiest lashes. Lancôme pumps tons of research into their mascaras—which are the best in the business—and this superstar is their bestseller.

Phytodefrisant: Plagued by frizz? Look no further than this plant-based miracle balm, which helps relax curls and waves, keeping locks sleek no matter *what* the humidity levels.

Lancôme Flash Bronzer Instant Colour Self-Tanning Leg Gel: The beauty editor favorite, as championed by industry legend (and, self-disclosure, my former boss) Jean Godfrey-June, who famously uses it everywhere, not just on legs. It gives "have you been at the beach?" color with a hint of shimmer, and looks natural—not orange—even in the dead of winter.

Yves Saint Laurent Touche Éclat Radiant Touch: Tired eyes? Suspicious shadows? Gone. YSL's cultiest product has light-reflecting particles to deflect attention from any unwanted spots or shadows while somehow—mysteriously, magically—brightening the entire face. Try it once, and you'll be hooked.

∽ BEAUTY CONFIDENTIAL: Getting in the Door

My first real interview was with the beauty director of one of the premiere magazines in the world. Allow me to set the scene for you. Me, a fresh-faced twenty-one-year-old college senior with three internships under my belt. She, the queen of the beauty industry and a woman who could make or break a brand with one line in her book. ("Book" is beauty editor lingo for a magazine.) In general, magazine offices do not look like a Kate Hudson or Jennifer Garner movie come to life, with assistants running about, photos of celebrities on the walls, and tasteful-yet-colorful décor.

Hers did. Two underlings sat at a desk outside her office in white shirts, smeared with red lipstick, examining shades as if the cure for cancer depended on it. As I cowered in my chair, facing her desk and an array of beauty products each more expensive than the cost of my outfit, ac-

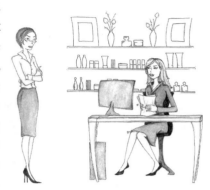

cessories, and haircut combined, I clutched my resumé tightly, wondering what the hell I was doing there. The meeting was blissfully sweet as she less interviewed me, more barked commands about what I *would* be expected to do ("You *will* show up promptly, call in all beauty products, conduct research, and liaise with publicists") and what I would *not* ("You will *not* call your boyfriend during office hours, play on instant messenger, check your personal emails, or waste my time."). I didn't get the job (surprise, surprise), but I did take away some valuable lessons from her. Number one: if you take yourself too seriously, you won't be winning any Miss Congeniality awards. Number two: if you take *beauty* too seriously, you suck all the fun out of it. And what's the point of that? (Now, in her case, it's her job, so I suppose it's actually to be commended that she and her staff approached it with such medical precision. It makes for a fabulous magazine, and a fabulous beauty section. I'm sure glad I didn't end up working there, though.)

THE LAZY GIRLS CLUB

Beauty editors are a fairly lazy bunch. We want pretty, we want chic, we want classic, we want impact—but above all, we want *fast*. Sure, we're willing to spend two hours in front of the mirror on a random Thursday evening recreating Jennifer Aniston's latest awards-show hairdo for the hell of it—but only, like, once a year. Otherwise? Speedy, please!

We're also not fashion editors. Fashion editors are—generally speaking, of course—perfectly turned out, impeccably coiffed, glossy, manicured, wearing threads that won't be available in the stores for months. Beauty editors? Let's just say that four-days-dirty hair, no makeup except for mascara and concealer, short, bare nails, and three-seasons-old clothing gifted by various beauty companies is the norm. Lest I make you think that all beauty editors are filthy, smelly hobos, let me assure you that's not the case. Beauty editors simply op-

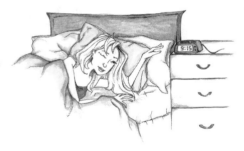

erate by the "less is more" maxim. Who has time to apply a full face of makeup, arrange a coiffed hairdo, coordinate a different outfit for every day of the week *and* be a fully functioning member of society? We're only human, after all! (Plus, beauty sleep is really, really important, and who wants to wake up early to doll yourself up when you could sleep in?)

When you've missed your alarm, or simply aren't feeling beauty motivated, here are the best tricks to get yourself out of the house in under ten minutes and still look great.

If you have only two minutes

▶ Great skin is the foundation of any look and is always the first thing you should address. (And, if you're pressed for time, is the *only* thing you should address.)

▶ If your skin is **perfect** (lucky you), apply a few swipes of light-reflecting concealer (with mica particles) around the eyes to brighten up the face.

▶ If your skin is **generally good**, with just a few imperfections, apply concealer to trouble spots.

▶ If your skin is more **troublesome**, with uneven tone and blemishes, apply foundation or tinted moisturizer with fingers (for a more natural look) to even out skin tone, then lightly add concealer as needed.

▶ No matter what your skin condition, finish with bronzer on your cheeks, temples, forehead, and brow bone. It will instantly warm up your face and give you a "done" look.

If you have only five minutes

▶ After you've "fixed" skin as directed above, the next most important thing is ensuring that eyes are defined.

▶ First, use an eyelash curler for five seconds on each lash.

▶ Next, take your mascara wand out of the tube and gently wipe it on a piece of tissue to remove excess product.

▶ Apply mascara to both the top and bottom of lashes, for extra definition (I like to apply mascara to the top first, then follow on the bottom to "spring" lashes back up).

If you have seven minutes

▶ Once your skin looks ready and your mascara is done, finish accentuating your eyes.

▶ Use your fingers to apply a sheer wash of peach, taupe, or copper eyeshadow from your eyelid to your browbone.

▶ Classic shades to try: Giorgio Armani Eyeshadow #12, Bobbi Brown eyeshadow in Bone, or NARS Eyeshadow in Nepal.

If you have ten minutes

▶ Skin? Check. Eyes? Check. Now it's time to warm up the rest of your face and complete the look.

▶ Lightly dust blush on the apples of your cheeks.

▶ NARS blush in Orgasm is killer (as we've already established), but you also might try NARS blush in Sin, Benefit Dandelion, MAC blush in Pinch O'Peach, or Jane Blushing Cheeks Powder Blush in Blushing Petal.

▶ Slick on a neutral, just-like-your-lips-but-even-better gloss such as Clinique Black Honey, Giorgio Armani Shine Gloss #4, or Stila lip pot in Mure.

▶ All finished! Subtle-yet-gorgeous in ten minutes flat. Not bad, eh?

❧ BEAUTY CONFIDENTIAL: A Day in the Life of a Beauty Editor

8:25 A.M.: Wakes up.

8:38 A.M.: Showers, not washing hair. (What's the need? She washed it two days ago and isn't due for another shampoo until tomorrow.)

8:56 A.M.: Throws on beauty editor uniform of jeans, flowy top, and trendy, feminine blazer. Briefly debates whether or not to wear a certain favorite shirt, then decides against it because there is an event today and the top was gifted by a public relations firm—which means every other editor has it, too.

8:59 A.M.: Slaps on SPF 30 tinted moisturizer, curls eyelashes, applies mascara, adds a few swipes of blush and lip gloss.

9:06 A.M.: Has a quick breakfast of nonfattening, skin-friendly foods—steel-cut oatmeal, blueberries, wild salmon, or egg whites.

9:19 A.M.: Out the front door.

9:46 A.M.: Arrives at work. Catches up on emails, phone messages, and office gossip. Opens first batch of publicist-sent beauty products and gifts. Moves to side of desk perfumes, body lotions, lip glosses, and makeup palettes she plans on taking home to "test." (Read: steal for herself and use . . . maybe eventually write about half.)

10:30 A.M.: Goes out to reception to greet first deskside of the day, where a mid-level publicist, marketing coordinator, and beauty executive will spend twenty minutes animatedly explaining why their (unfortunately) unexceptional product is in fact *extremely* exceptional. Nods and smiles politely while silently wondering if her beauty lunch event will feature actual food this time, or just blueberries and salmon like last time.

10:56 A.M.: Gets back to desk, where another delivery of beauty products from companies and publicity firms is waiting. Score! It's the new, limited-edition Marc Jacobs perfume that she surreptitiously called in yesterday evening, whispering into the phone that it was for an upcoming story . . . which it's not.

11:30 A.M.: Receives an orchid, live goldfish, or box of chocolates from a publicist thanking her for last month's article.

11:55 A.M.: Remembers she has a beauty lunch cross-town in five minutes, grabs purse, rushes out the door frantically, fixes hair and makeup to look presentable in the waiting town car (called by the company throwing the event, natch).

12:13 P.M.: Arrives breathlessly, throwing apologies everywhere. Looks around, realizes she is only the fifth editor to arrive and everybody else is, in fact, running later than she was.

12:30 P.M.: Event starts half an hour late. Chats quietly with other editors while eating salmon and blueberries, taking notes on the presentation (latest skincare advances) and wondering what the hell is up with that associate editor's outfit over there in the corner.

2:05 P.M.: Cheek-kisses editors and publicists as departs with goody bag in tow. Paws through bag in cab, excited to discover that it not only contains full-sized samples of the promising new line, but also a two-hundred-dollar gift card to Barneys. Awesome! Being a beauty editor is *so* worth it.

2:28 P.M.: Arrives back at office, spends the next hour and a half writing upcoming article, taking only short breaks to occasionally read Gawker and open new deliveries of beauty products.

3:50 P.M.: Calls publicists to request products for upcoming article. Stresses that they need to "rush" them over, because she's "way past deadline."

4:05 P.M.: Flips through the new issues of *Allure* and *Vogue*, dog-earing articles to read in detail later. Tears out a few ads of models and celebrities with really, really good hair and tacks them to her bulletin board for inspiration.

4:15 P.M.: Secretly wishes she smoked so that she could take random ten-minute breaks four times a day like the people in the art department.

4:17 P.M.: Freaks out when assistant nervously reveals that she accidentally lost the bag filled with ten "comp" bottles of perfume from last month's story. Insists that the assistant calls the companies herself to break the news. Wonders for the seventy-fifth time why publicists and beauty executives get so worked up over those stupid glass mock-up bottles, which they insist cost "thousands of dollars." Wishes again she smoked. Thinks of the free-radicals this would cause, briefly feels both calmer and prettier.

4:30 P.M.: Interviews world-famous makeup artist over the phone about the best ways to create a smoky-eye.

5:05 P.M.: Spends twenty minutes going through products on desk, looking for new beauty trends for next week's memo. Puts more products in a bag to bring home and test, making mental note to call in duplicates tomorrow.

5:25 P.M.: Quickly touches up makeup and hair, adding eyeliner, bronzer and more lip gloss, puts on spare pair of heels she keeps under desk and heads out the door to evening beauty event.

6:03 P.M.: Arrives downtown for the launch of a new celebrity-backed perfume. Heads straight for the open bar, orders the specialty cocktail, then spends the next two hours chatting with other beauty girls, and gobbling up hors d'oeuvres from the trays circulated by hot model waiters. Briefly meets the celebrity in question, marvels at A) how much prettier in person she is (as if that's even possible) or B) how much of an inarticulate airhead she is (as if that's even a surprise).

8:30 P.M.: Heads home in a town car armed with a beauty bag stuffed to the brim with loot: the new perfume, a copy of the celebrity's latest DVD or CD, a small pair of diamond earrings, and the latest iPod. Marvels at how she has the coolest, strangest job in the world.

∿ Beauty Secret

Some beauty products and services are worth it. Some aren't. Beauty editors quickly learn what falls into what category.

WHAT TO SPLURGE ON

Eyeshadow: The more finely milled powders in prestige eyeshadows (great brands: Dior, Chanel, Lancôme, MAC) equal longer wear and less creasing. Buy a few staple shades that you'll wear every day and which will carry you from boardroom to bedroom, and then save the nighttime-and-party-shade experimentation for the drugstore.

Concealer: Cheap concealers simply don't cover up shadows, hide imperfections, or last as long. They're also more likely to crease, which will give you that lovely melting-wax look that's so hot nowadays.

Conditioner: While there are scores of excellent conditioners available at drug and specialty stores (some with nearly identical ingredients to pricier brands—see Chapter Two), there's no denying that an effective conditioner makes a world of difference on hair, especially hair that's coarse, frizzy, or damaged. If you've tried various cheapie conditioners but can't help coming back to your old, more expensive favorite, don't feel guilty. You just have fussy hair, dahling.

Haircut: I can't stress this enough: a good haircut is crucial. Keep searching until you find a stylist you love, and if it's more expensive than you can afford, extend your time between cuts.

Hair Tools: When you're dealing with several hundred degrees of heat on your hair, you'd better make sure the apparatus is the highest-quality, most evenly heated one you can find. Unless you use your styling tools only a few times a year, the money you save now will be wasted later on treatments for your split ends and tissues for your tears.

Highlights: Hair is so demanding, isn't it? There's a plethora of drugstore, DIY highlighting kits available now, but I'd advise you to use at your own risk. For every success story I've heard (which would be zero), I've seen literally dozens of haircolor tragedies. If orange streaks are your thing, have fun—otherwise leave it to the pros.

Pedicures: Manicures are easy to do at home when you know the proper tricks. Pedicures, on the other hand, are often more trouble than they're worth, and can be difficult to make look salon-professional. Get a salon pedicure once a month, then just change the polish yourself every week or two (or three!) if you can't afford the regular upkeep.

THINGS TO GET FOR CHEAP

Fragrance: Now, I'm not exactly advocating cheap perfume. I, personally, can't stand many of the lower-end scents on the market. But fragrance is a very personal thing . . . and what smells cheap on me might smell like gold on you. Before she created her popular scent Lovely, Sarah Jessica Parker was known to wear musk oil that she bought for years at the drugstore. And when I was at *Lucky*, several of the editors confessed to a shameful addiction: Glow by J. Lo, which may not be bargain-bin, but is hardly Clive Christian. The bottom line? If you find a scent that you love, and which smells fabulous on you, wear it proudly—no matter what the price tag.

Cleanser: It's on your skin for less than a minute and then slides down the drain, so what's the point of paying big bucks for a designer cleanser? Save the money and spend it instead on an effective moisturizer—with ingredients that'll penetrate and remain on your face all day.

Nail polish: It always amazes me how otherwise intelligent, sane women are willing to shell out, say, forty bucks for a nail polish that is actually inferior to other brands, simply because it has a designer label. (So not naming names here.) In fact, some of the best-quality nail polishes are available at the drugstore, such as Rimmel, Sally Hansen, and Revlon. My personal favorite brand, Essie, is also a relative bargain at about $14, and the fabulousness that is OPI only costs around $7. There are some things you need a designer label for. Nail polish—which, let's face it, chips inside of a week no matter *what* brand you buy, or how much top coat you slap on it—is not one of them.

Moisturizer: While it's true that you get what you pay for—and that an effective moisturizer chock full of skin-boosting ingredients such as glycolic acid, retinol, or antioxidants is the quickest and easiest way to keep your skin clear, smooth and glowing—there's simply no reason to spend hundreds of dollars on a moisturizer when you can find one nearly as good (or in some cases, even better!) at the drugstore. Many top drugstore beauty companies spend millions on research, meaning you'll find the same technology at your local CVS as you would at Neiman Marcus. The packaging may not be as glamorous, and the name not as exciting, but at the end of the day, your skin won't know the difference. (In fact, a recent independent study comparing several high-end moisturizers with their drugstore counterparts named Olay Regenerist the best . . . outshining anti-aging creams literally five times more expensive.)

PRODUCTS TO BRING BACK FROM EUROPE

What is it about European products that makes us (okay, well, maybe just me) open my wallet as wide as it will allow, frantically snapping up products as if I'd never before seen shampoo, moisturizer, or candles? It's the thrill of the unknown, as well as the glamour factor that comes from proudly displaying an exotic-looking bottle on your vanity, with all of the writing in Italian, French, German, or Spanish (eh, just 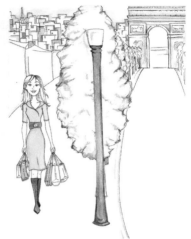 insert your favorite high school language here), with the fantasy that an old acquaintance of yours might pop by the house, wander into your bathroom, see the array of foreign beauty products, and exclaim, "My God! I never knew you were so worldly! No *wonder* you always look gorgeous!" That's the hope, right? Of course, aesthetics and fancy labels only take you so far. The reason the following products are beloved by beauty editors, experts, and world travelers alike is because, quite simply, they *work*. Some are easily bought in boutique drugstores in New York and Los Angeles, but are not as easy to find in other parts of the country. So next time you're taking that business trip to London, or honeymoon to Paris (I'm sure your new hubby won't mind), swing by the local beauty emporium and pick up these gems:

England

L'Oreal Elnett hairspray: A light hold, guaranteed-to-find-it-in-every-single-professional-hairstylist's-kit favorite, this aerosol is easy to brush out, not-too-sticky, and perfect for when you don't want anybody to know that you're actually wearing hairspray.

Jemma Kidd Makeup School Lasting Tint Semi-Permanent Waterproof Mascara: Created by English fashion model-turned makeup artist Jemma Kidd, this hint-of-color, lasts-for-days mascara is perfect for those times (like, say, a camping trip with a new guy) when you need to look naturally pretty but can't spend any time making yourself up. The rest of the line, with clear, easy-to-use instructions, is pretty fabulous, too.

Louise Galvin Sacred Locks: With no preservatives or synthetic ingredients, London-based celebrity colorist Louise Galvin's hair care line is designed to revive damaged, fragile, colored hair and nourish it back to life. The cult of Sacred Locks products is slavish, indeed (and for good reason).

Italy

Santa Maria Novella: A centuries-old apothecary run by monks in a church in Florence, these goodies are the very definition of Italian glamour. With everything from perfumes commissioned by Catherine de Medici (try Ambra or Acqua di Colonia) to medicinal elixirs to body oils, the products are still produced by monks, and are not only guaranteed to impress aforementioned bathroom visitors, but are also deliciously decadent to use.

Portugal

Claus Porto: The best, most giftable soaps ever—not to mention adored the world over for more than a hundred years—these are less like body products and more like delectable treats, in flavors like Wild Pansy, Red Poppy, and

Honeysuckle and wrapped in such divine, visually stunning packaging that it's almost a crime to open and actually *use* them.

Germany

Dr Hauschka: A holistic, plant-based, ecologically responsible skin-care line that doesn't test on animals and uses as many organic ingredients as possible, beloved by Madonna and those who are just as concerned about what they put on their bodies as they are about what they put in them.

France

La Roche Posay Anthelios XL: The *ne plus ultra* of sun protection, this product is virtually worshipped as a skin saver. To say that it's considered the best sunscreen in the world is not an overstatement.

Diptyque candles: There's a candle . . . and then there's a Diptyque candle. With a price tag more akin to a bottle of expensive perfume, the many scents in this lush line are just as rewarding as an expert fragrance creation from Grasse. It's hard to pick only one, but my favorite is the ever-popular blackcurrant-and-Bulgarian-rose-infused Baies.

BEAUTY MYTH: *French Women Are Inherently Prettier, Sexier, and More Chic Than You. Oh. And They Don't Get Fat Either.*

Is Brigitte Bardot to blame? Catherine Deneuve? That cute chick from *Amelie* and *The Da Vinci Code*? I'm not here to point fingers, but simply to call a spade a spade. You, my friend, were born under an unlucky star. Why, you ask? Simple. Because you're not French. French women, you see, have more sex appeal, more style, more *je ne sais quoi* (the decks are *so* stacked in their favor on that one, by the way, seeing as the expression comes from their native language and all) in their pinky fingers than you do in your entire Yankee-born and bred, apple-pie-loving, *American Idol*-watching body. It's not a subjective observation. It's a *fact*. I mean, it must be, seeing as there are endless books devoted to it. And, it's pretty much impossible to open up a woman's magazine of a certain caliber without finding an article titled "Secrets of the French," or "Ooh La La! Beauty tips from France," or, like, "American Women Should All Just Give Up and Move to Paris, Otherwise You're Destined For a Life of Ugliness." Don't get me wrong—I love France. I refused to call them "Freedom Fries" a few years back; I studied in Paris during college; I cite my high-school exchange student as inarguable proof that there are seriously delightful French people in this world. But the notion that French women are born better, more beautiful and more stylish than you and me? Rubbish. (I mean, no offense to them . . . but have you *been* to France? Have you *seen* some of the dowdy, clunky-soled, black-nyloned, tweedy-skirted, Queen-Elizabeth-in-the-garden-with-the-dogs outfits they've got going on? Sure, the women are chic on the Avenue Montaigne, but privileged women in a small district does not an entire nation of fashionistas make.) What's really going on here is that most of the magazine editors are in love with Paris and the romance that clings to it—not to mention the idealized version of French women they encounter once a year in the City of Lights during the couture shows. Plus, it's an easy way to toss off a four-page piece without really trying, since the theory is pretty much accepted as gospel by the entire beauty world. Hey! Let's write a magazine article about it! We'll stuff it with pretty pictures of gorgeous French celebs (of whom there are many . . . but what about Scarlett Johansson, Jennifer Aniston, Cindy Crawford, Aisha Tyler, Grace Kelly, Demi Moore, Diane Sawyer, Tyra Banks, Lana Turner, Diane Lane, Beverly Johnson, Marilyn Monroe, Christy Turlington, Vanessa Williams, Jennifer Lopez, Rita Hayworth, Kelly Hu, Sharon Stone . . . need I continue?), add some good quotes *en Francais,* and throw a catchy title on it. *Voila!* And that's how a soul crushing, nation-bashing trend is born. *Vive la revolution de maquillage!*

Direct from Jolie in NYC

I get emailed certain questions over and over to answer on my blog. Here, a real question from a real reader, with my real response. (It's all so real.)

Q: *I was hoping you could offer some advice. I'm a recent college graduate, not much younger than yourself, and contemplating a possible future in magazines, specifically those dealing with fashion/beauty/all the usual suspects. I went to a good school and finished with a degree in journalism. Writing for a magazine, rather working my way up to a writing position, is always something else I wanted to do. Any advice how to get a chance doing this though I don't have the internship experience, etc.? Or any advice to steer clear of this? I just know you worked your way up the ladder at a young age and it is inspiring and makes me somewhat hopeful if this is what I choose to do. I appeciate your listening (er, reading) . . .*

A: Okay, here goes: Getting a job in the magazine industry without internships is tough. I wish that weren't the case, but people are 99% of the time simply unwilling to take a chance on somebody unproven . . . even if it's for something as simple as answering phones and opening packages! In an ideal world, you'd have racked up internships during college, since most internships are unpaid and must be taken for college credit—unfair, huh? If, at the present time, you can't get an internship (either because nobody will hire you or you simply can't afford it), make friends with somebody who works at a magazine. Unfortunately, it's still about who you know, and having a friend "on the inside" who can alert you to assistant openings is key. Find a mid-level editor whose work you admire and email her to ask if she'll let you treat her to coffee. Bring your resume, spend twenty minutes or half an hour picking her brain, and then check in every so often to see if she's heard of any openings or has any advice. You'll be pleasantly surprised—most women in the industry will go out of their way to help you, often because somebody did the same for them. And finally, don't be afraid to stalk the HR people at the big magazine companies (you can find their numbers on *Ed2010.com*) until they agree to set up an informational interview. Following the informational, call once a month just to check in and see if any positions have opened. Some might disagree with this, but HR reps are only people, after all (not monsters!), and I know many, many people (including myself with my first post-college position) who have scored jobs this way. Finally, check out *Ed2010.com* and *Mediabistro.com* daily. It will probably take a few months (maybe as long as a year), but if you're persistent and passionate, you will eventually find something great that will, down the road, lead to something even better. Good luck!

∽ BEAUTY CONFIDENTIAL: Learning to grow up and stop being a swag hag

When I whispered on my blog about the orgy of free designer goods sent to beauty editors, I was simply marveling at the fact, not complaining about it or trying to take down the industry. (Trust me.) Who knew a job existed where you're paid to write about lipstick and get free haircuts and visit chichi spas *gratis* and have a bathroom rivaling Sephora *and* receive free Marc Jacobs and Chanel and Louis Vuitton everything as gifts at Christmastime? Uh . . . who *wouldn't* like that?

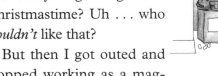

But then I got outed and stopped working as a magazine editor and started focusing at the time on other stuff (freelancing, my blog, my books, *Laguna Beach*). I still received beauty products to test and write about, though of course not with the same frequency as before—when you're getting between twenty and thirty bags a day filled to the brim with shampoo, candles, and eye shadow, anything less, even while still an embarrassment of riches, pales in comparison. But once I started working at home and didn't have an office—or a beauty closet—to store everything in, I couldn't have handled many more products, anyway. That's fine. I'm stocked with conditioner and foundation and moisturizer for the next four years or so.

It's the purses I miss.

Ahh, the purses. Every week, a new bag, smartly wrapped from a chipper PR exec and more often than not accompanied by a relevant product. Orange essence facial cleanser? Here! Try some, and while you're at it, here's an orange Longchamp bag to go with it! Sick of dry skin when you fly? Try our miracle moisturizing balm, perfect for long, arid flights. Oh, hell, while you're at it, take this DVF travel bag, too! Tired of reviewing beauty products? You *have* had an awfully long year. Here's a Rafe purse, with our compliments. Love ya! Write about us!

Several years of working in the industry has provided me with a varied and numerous array of duffle bags, L.L. Bean totes, wristlets, clutches, hobos, overnighters, and shoulder bags. I really don't need to buy another purse . . . well . . . ever. But how do you go from all to nothing? "How will I survive Christmas without a fresh supply of totes (and scarves and wallets and sunglasses, too)?" I thought. Oh, cruel world that rains Gucci upon you and then suddenly yanks it all away!

Then I realized, um, it's just stuff. And I started focusing on more important things, like, mmm, writing—and the very thing I was *meant* to be focusing on, which was beauty, of course. Silly me.

Chapter One Product Price Guide

$: less than $10
$$: between $10 and $24
$$$: between $25 and $49
$$$$: between $50 and $100
$$$$$: more than $100

NARS blush in Orgasm, $$$, *narscosmetics.com*
Terax Crema, $$, *sephora.com*
Essie Mademoiselle, $, *essiecosmetics.com*
OPI I'm Not Really a Waitress, $, *opi.com*
Mario Badescu Drying Potion, $$, *mariobadescu.com*
Shu Uemura Eyelash Curler, $$, *shuuemura-usa.com*
Bumble and bumble Does It All Styling Spray, $$,
   bumbleandbumble.com for locations
Cetaphil Face Wash, $, drugstores
Kiehl's Lip Balm # 1, $, *kiehls.com*
Lancôme Definicils, $$, *lancôme-usa.com*
Phytodefrisant, $$$, *phyto-usa.com*
**Lancôme Flash Bronzer Instant Colour Self-Tanning Leg
   Gel,** $$$, *lancome-usa.com*
Yves Saint Laurent Touche Éclat Radiant Touch, $$$,
   nordstrom.com
Giorgio Armani Eyeshadow #12, $$$,
   giorgioarmanibeauty-usa.com for locations
Bobbi Brown Eyeshadow in Bone, $$, *bobbibrowncosmetics.com*
NARS Eyeshadow in Nepal, $$, *sephora.com*
NARS blush in Sin, $$, *sephora.com*

Benefit Dandelion, $$, *benefitcosmetics.com*
Mac Pinch O'Peach, $$, *maccosmetics.com*
Jane Blushing Cheeks Powder Blush in Blushing Petal, $,
    drugstores
Clinique Black Honey, $$, *clinique.com*
Giorgio Armani Shine Gloss #4, $$,
    giorgioarmanibeauty-usa.com for locations
Stila Lip Pot in Mure, $$, *stila.com*
Dior eye shadow, $$$, *eluxury.com*
Chanel eye shadow, $$$, *chanel.com*
Lancôme eye shadow, $$$, *Lancômeusa.com*
MAC eyeshadow, $$$, *maccosmetics.com*
Sarah Jessica Parker Lovely, $$$, *sarahjessicaparkerbeauty.com*
Glow by J.Lo, $$$, *shopjlo.com*
Clive Christian, $$$$$, *neimanmarcus.com, saksfifthavenue.com*
Rimmel, $, drugstores
Sally Hansen polish, $, drugstores
Revlon nail polish, $, drugstores
Essie nail polish, $, *essie.com* for locations
Olay Regenerist, $$, drugstores
L'oreal Elnett hairspray, $$, *zitomer.com*
**Jemma Kidd Makeup School Lasting Tint Semi-Permanent
    Waterproof Mascara,** $$$, *neimanmarcus.com*
Santa Maria Novella, $$, *lafcony.com*
Claus Porto, $$, *lafcony.com*
Dr Hauschka, $$$, *drhauschka.com*
La Roche Posay Anthelios XL, $$$, *zitomer.com*
Diptyque candles, $$$, *neimanmarcus.com*

Two

Hairstyling

Hairdressers that make love to your hair . . .
and other adventures in styling

When it comes to that all-important client-stylist relationship, I am a horrendous failure. In movies, the fabulous woman breezes into the salon, lobbing kisses right and left as she spies Olivier or Roberto or whomever her equally *gorge* stylist happens to be. He trims, she confides in him whatever plagues her at the moment, and champagne is sipped by all. Bonds are formed. Beauty happens.

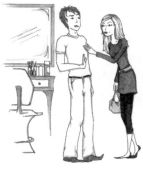

My client-stylist interactions usually involve me arriving at the salon fifteen minutes late, having inevitably been stuck in traffic, then awkwardly going in for a kiss with my stylist as he tries to give me a hug. I don't know what it is about me, but I rarely cultivate those kiss-kiss "Darling!" relationships with my stylists. I try to confide. I try to gossip. It rarely works. I saw one particular stylist for two years and kept crawling back despite the slightly chilly reception I felt he always gave me. I finally gathered the courage to leave him when he called me by the wrong name. I broke it off with another when, despite my gentle but repeated protestations that "I have a really sensitive scalp," he insisted on pulling and tugging my hair while shampooing, combing, and blow-drying it, often to the point where I was biting my lip to keep from squealing in pain.

No doubt about it, going to the salon can be a harrowing experience.

In my mind, however, worse than the cold, aloof stylists who couldn't give a crap about you (hey, at least you can sit in peace and read your magazine) are the ones who are too, shall we say, hot. If you've never had the privilege of the stylist who makes love to your hair, you're missing out. You sit in the chair and he immediately plunges his hands into your tresses, stroking your scalp, winding his fingers through your strands, leaning close and murmuring in your ear what he wants to do to you: "A little fringe . . . some layers in the back . . . ohh . . . so sexy . . . so sexy." After he finishes shampooing (Oh, lord, the shampooing!), cutting, and blow-drying, he goes back for seconds, fondling your head again while flipping hair this way and that, until he's convinced he's achieved the perfect look guaranteed to turn the head of every male within a five-mile radius. It's kind of embarrassing the first time and entertaining the second, but by the third, it just gets old. You start to worry: Is he straight? Is he attracted to me? Should I start wearing makeup to the salon? Am I getting a zit? What if he's gay? Is he just doing it for a bigger tip? When I go to the salon, I want to relax, forget all my worries, and concentrate on the fact that I'm going to leave looking one hundred times better than I did when I walked in, not feel like I have to avoid looking Jean-Pierre in the eyes for fear of having him slobber on my neck.

It took me years of trial and error, experimentation, and variety to find my current stylists and colorists, who've been with me through long and short, blond and black, and everything in between. (Kristin Vincelli and Kathy Galotti at Louis Licari salon, I salute you!) When you finally find that special stylist, it's nirvana. But even at your favorite salon, it's easy to feel unsure about the simplest things, such as who and what to tip. Here, a cheat sheet so that you're never stuck at the salon again.

✺ Tipping

In general, 20% of the service price is a good bet, with a few exceptions.

Shampoo girl: For a fancy salon, five to ten dollars is standard; two or three dollars is perfectly acceptable at your garden-variety salon. If you forget to tip her, while nobody will shoot you evil glares or ban you from the salon on your next visit, it *is* considered slightly rude. Tip extra the next time to make up for it.

Blow out: If you're at the salon solely for a blowout or style, with no other services scheduled, tip 20% of the total cost. If the blowout is included in your color or cut, and performed by somebody other than your stylist, such as her assistant, tipping between five and fifteen dollars will be appreciated.

Haircutter/stylist: Always give your stylist at least 20%, never less. Feel free to tip more, of course, if you're over the moon about the modern-mullet or pixie-crop or Gisele-layers (or whatever) she gave you. But be aware, if you tip badly, the stylist *will* remember on your next visit. (Not to put the fear of God in you, but I'm just saying . . .)

Colorist: While a lot of hard work obviously goes into cutting hair, I always save my biggest and best tips for my colorist. Not only does this procedure take the longest, but, in my mind, it's the hardest to get right, so good work deserves a fantastic reward. Again, 20% is standard, but I usually give my colorist 25% or 30%. (In return, she sometimes throws in a free glaze or treatment on my next visit—and then everybody's happy.)

And all the rest: Don't forget the girl who gave you tea, the woman who checked your coat, and your stylist's assistant! 1% or 2% is fine, or about two or three dollars each.

Celebrity-stylist Mark Garrison on tipping

"Good service deserves to be recognized. Just like a restaurant, a salon is a service industry, and it's expected you will acknowledge those who have assisted you. Giving 15 to 20 percent of the cost of your service is an average tip; it demonstrates that you like what you had done and are happy. A tip over 20 percent shows more appreciation for that awesome job you really love. Acknowledge all those who assist you at the salon—and they will remember you kindly on all your return visits."

∾ Salon Etiquette

Okay, so you've saved the money, thought of appropriate fibs to tell your significant other about how much it will cost ("Where did that $200 go? I paid off the credit card—I swear!"), and have booked an appointment at Vincent-

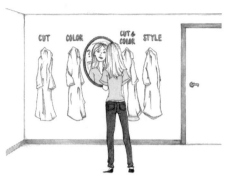

Maxime's House of Fabulous Styles For the Rich and Chic. Your first time in a fancy salon can be a bit nervewracking, however, especially if you're the type who worries about saying the right things, tipping appropriately and just generally trying not to make an ass out of yourself. Fret not. *You're* paying *them*, and it should be a morning or afternoon of fun and relaxation, not discomfort and nervousness. It may seem elementary, but I'll guide you through it anyway.

▶ Wear one of your favorite outfits, so the stylist can see you in your "regular" clothes.

▶ Arrive and let the person at the check-in desk know you're there.

▶ Wait to be led into the changing room. Often, you'll be asked what kind of service you're having by an attendant. This is because some salons provide different colored robes, based on whether you're just having a cut, or are also having a color service such as highlights.

▸ Take off your shirt, leave on your bra, and put on the robe. You might feel uncomfortable and want to leave your shirt on, but it's best to disrobe, as you don't want hairs all over your shirt later—or, worse, peroxide.

▸ Put your shirt on a hanger and give it to the attendant. If there is no attendant, leave your shirt hanging in the changing room. An assistant will come and hang it up for you.

▸ Go back out to the waiting area until called by your stylist. If it's a multi-level salon, ask at the front desk which floor your services are on, head to that floor, and then check in with reception. They'll lead you to a chair to await your stylist.

▸ Bring a picture for your stylist, to minimize confusion about what look you're after. (Even better, bring looks of styles you *don't* want.)

▸ If you're not a talkative type, feel free to zone out, read a magazine, or stay silent while your stylist is working. Make sure to keep your head level, however, so your stylist can best cut and style your head. (A stylist once reprimanded me for crossing my legs while he cut, claiming this resulted in an uneven chop. Whether it was true or not, I now keep my legs uncrossed.)

▸ Speak up in the shampoo chair—if you have a sensitive scalp or the water is too hot or cold, say so! Trust me, they won't like you more just because you sat biting your lip while all your hair was ripped out.

▸ Ask your stylist questions as they work. Curious about why they're snipping here or shearing there? Wondering what the best way to style your hair will be? Interested in their take on the differences between drugstore and prestige haircare products? Ninety-nine times out of a hundred, the stylist will be thrilled to share her expertise with you.

▶ Change back into your street clothes before tipping, so your stylist has a chance to see the finished results.

▶ If you're shy about tipping or saying goodbye, simply thank the stylist for her work as you leave her chair, then place the tip in an envelope with her name written on top (I like to add a short, personal note of thanks) and hand it to the receptionist.

And what about if you'd rather poke your eyes out than be forced to carry on an inane conversation with your stylist? (Hey, it happens.) Is it rude to pull out a magazine, you wonder, or are you required to chat politely under pain of death (and bad haircut)? As it turns out, most stylists don't care. (Seriously.) As long as your head is positioned wherever they'd like it for maximum cutting/highlighting/styling, they really couldn't give a flip. So there you go.

∾ BEAUTY MYTH: A $25 cut looks the same as a $250 cut

Wouldn't it be nice if this were true? Sadly, it's not. Nearly always, the stylist charging $250 for a cut is truly worth her salt and *deserves* to be charging that much because she's worked her way up the salon food chain and has put in years of training with the best names in the business. The stylist charging $25, while perhaps no less naturally talented (hey, you never know), simply doesn't have access to the same level of expertise, training, and experience. If she did, she'd audition for a top-level salon, work her way up to a head stylist job, and start making bank. And then *she'd* start charging $250 for a cut, too. Stylist differences aside, more expensive cuts tend to grow out better, look more natural (as if your hair just "happens" to fall oh-so-perfectly like that) and cut down on your styling time. Your haircut is the foundation of your entire look, and it's something that you have to live with every single day. Is there a difference between, say, a $60 cut and one that's $120? That's for you to decide. You can find phenomenal drugstore shampoos, conditioners, and styling products. But when it comes to the cut itself, I take no chances. (Oribe, the celebrity stylist who charges about $800 per cut, with some of the most magic hands in the business, cites the famous MasterCard commercials. "A bad cut equals months of fighting with your hair and unhappiness in your appearance. A good, easy-to-style cut? Priceless.")

> *Some of the worst mistakes of my life have been haircuts.*
>
> *Jim Morrison*

∾ The Power of Great Hair

Have you ever exited the salon with a haircut that you weren't crazy about and run home crying to your husband or boyfriend, only to have him say, "Relax. It's just hair"? Have you then wanted to stab him in the thigh with a dull fork? Yes? Okay, good, we're on the same page. A fantastic haircut can redefine your image, help you get over a bad relationship, attract a new one, and, of course, instill a much-deserved sense of confidence in your appearance. (These claims are not overblown, by the way. I can't count the number of times my friends and I have made huge, symbolic hair changes as a successful way of letting go of past traumas in our lives.) A bad cut, on the other hand ... is there anything worse? Maybe death, poverty, disease, and ... nope, that's about it. A celebrity like Madonna has realized the power that can come with hair reinvention: long and black? Hey, she's kinda Indian! Short and curly? Why, hey, there, Marilyn! Sleek, chic, rich-bitch-blond chignon? It's Eva Peron herself! Jennifer Aniston is another example of a celeb who makes the most of her hair. I love Jennifer. I think she's adorable. But the girl is *all* hair. When she dyes it super-dark, scrapes it back tightly off her face, or appears with it wet (as she did in her nude scene in *The Break Up*), she's no longer a beautiful, sexy goddess. She's just ... a cute girl with a sort of pointy chin and blue eyes. So, what does she do? She wears her hair long and proud, with variations of the same highlights over and over and over and over. And it doesn't just look good on her—it's *fabulous* on her. The point? Learn what works for you, and pimp it like it's going out of style. If you get bored with the same style for more than a few months, go crazy: dye it, cut it, get extensions, curl it, hell, get a Mohawk, if that's your thing. Conversely, if you've had your hair in roughly the same style for the past decade—not because you're afraid of change, but because that's honestly the perfect look for you—then don't feel pressured to change it simply to rock the boat. (And you'd be in good company—Anna Wintour has been clinging to that short brown bob practically since I was born, and she looks amazing.) After all, pretty is pretty.

∽ How To: Create the Perfect Ponytail

The perfect ponytail, much like the perfect man, is something of a myth. (Does it really exist? Do you know anybody who actually has one? Have you seen one in *real life*?) Rest assured, it is indeed out there, my friends. (Well, the perfect ponytail, at least. Jury's still out on the man thing.) It takes a little experimentation, and a lot of trial and error to find one that matches your personal style, but I've seen the promised land. And it looks good.

You've probably heard that updos work best on dirty hair. This is true in every occasion *except* with the ponytail. A ponytail is best on squeaky-clean hair. Otherwise, it just looks dirty and messy, like you're on your way back from the gym. For a truly stylin' pony, wash and dry your hair, taking care to style it as sleekly as possible. (This may or may not involve straightening shampoos and flatirons.)

There are now two options: the chic low pony, cinched at the nape of your neck; or the pony gathered a few inches below your crown. In general, if you are above the age of eighteen and not a high-school cheerleader, you should avoid the high ponytail tied at your crown as a style statement. (Unless, of course, you are being ironic or heading to a Halloween party. Then, by all means.)

For the chic low ponytail, part your hair deeply on one side, then brush it smoothly over across your forehead. Tuck any stray pieces behind your ear or mist with hairspray. (The key to this look is the hair framing your eyes. Add a bit of smudgy black eyeliner for extra drama.) Keep the hair sleek and close to your head, pulling it back and securing at the nape of your neck.

For the ponytail gathered a few inches below your crown, the trick is to add volume at the top of your head, either by teasing it, or by attaching a few small temporary extensions for volume. (Danilo

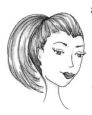

and Ken Paves make high-quality but relatively inexpensive pieces you can have fun with and use for nights out. Just keep in mind, your boyfriend will probably hate them. Most boys tend to have a thing about not finding fake hair sexy. Go figure.) Put your fingers at the crown of your head and gather up a large section of hair, about three inches wide by two inches deep, teasing it on the underneath to create volume. Run your hairbrush over this section lightly, then pull hair into a ponytail just above the middle point at the back of your head. This look is most chic when secured with a hair-covered elastic, or when you wrap a strand of your hair around the elastic itself, pinning underneath the ponytail with a bobby pin. If your hair needs more volume, place your palms on the top of your head and slowly, gently, slide them up, pulling the back of your hair ever so slightly up while keeping it secured in the elastic. Finish with a light misting on hairspray, concentrating on the sides and back of hair.

∿ Change Your Look in Three Seconds Flat

Change your part, and you'll change your life. Okay, this is a slight exaggeration, but if you belong to the school of good hair = happiness, nothing shakes up your look faster than a dramatic part change. Normally wear your hair all flippy and coquettish and surfer girl, with no discernable part? Take a comb and draw a deep part on the side of your head, with your bangs or front part of your hair lying low across your forehead and tucked behind your ear. Addicted to side parts? Try a center part, which—despite what some of you may think—*can* work on non-oval face shapes, as long as you have enough volume (think Brigitte Bardot–messy). And if you've been wearing your hair parted on the right for the last eight years, you'll be amazed at the volume and lift that you'll get from switching it to the left (or vice versa).

∿ The Different Hairstylists

Gay Psychiatrist: He's gay. He's chatty. He's empathetic. And he's *fabulous*. This is the kind of stylist who always pops up in movies as Reese or Julia's mane man, designed to both whip your locks into shape and sagely explain why your boyfriend is a total idiot. Except he's not only in movies—he's real. After twenty-five minutes in his chair, he'll know the name of your last three exes, the fact that your second cousin got a girl pregnant, and the *real* reason your best friend stopped talking to you for two weeks in 2003. He's your soulmate. If only he were straight. Well, at least he gives great cut.

The European Lover: Have you ever had a stylist stare deeply into your eyes while caressing your scalp, whispering amorously that he is going to make your hair *perfect*? If so, you've been struck by the European Lover. Without fail, he's either French or Italian, and usually speaks English with a heavy (but oh-so-sexy) accent. He'll ply you with compliments, immediately inquire whether you have a boyfriend, and seduce your hair with his hands. Before your next appointment, you'll spend ten extra minutes applying makeup, because how could Claude possibly see you without it? Your hopes will be dashed, however, when his much older girlfriend Barbara shows up at the salon. These relationships, much like real ones, often last only a year or two before one of you loses interest because of the lack of sex.

The Style Nazi: Every time you come in, he seems to take perverse pleasure in pointing out how bad your hair looks, how you've damaged it, how the style is all wrong, and in generally beating your self-esteem into the ground. Then he explains how *he* is the only stylist in the world who can fix it. The Style

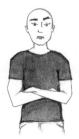

Nazi is usually all the more annoying because he will give you the most fantastic cut of your life, and you will receive compliments every day for two weeks. When you leave him (probably for a confidence-bolstering Gay Psychiatrist or European Lover), your mother will complain each time you see her that your hair does not look as good as it used to.

The Bored Stylist: This is the stylist who seems to wish that he were anywhere but with *you*. Whether it's chatting with the assistant (and shooting you nasty glances when you try to participate in the conversation), talking on the phone with his best friend about how terrible his day has been so far, or sighing loudly as he snips and stares into space, this hairstylist makes it clear that you are his very last priority. The only thing more insulting than the Bored 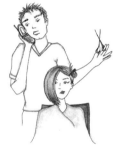 Stylist is when the Bored Stylist's next client arrives at the salon early and receives hugs, kisses, and chatty enquiries about how the kids are—in the middle of *your* cut.

∾ How To: Give yourself a salon-worthy blowout

What is the most annoying thing in the world? Nails on a blackboard? Little old ladies driving thirty miles under the speed limit in the left lane? Teenaged girls roaming the malls in packs of ten, ignoring each other as they yap on their cell phones while wearing clothes that would make hookers blush? Annoying all, but no, no, and no. It is, in case you weren't aware, the fact that it is *literally impossible* to blow-dry your hair anywhere near as well as your hairdresser does. I don't know what kind of magical powers their arms and hands have, because I can replicate my salon experience to a T—I mean, we're talking same blow-dryer, same brushes, same products, same ridiculously long length of time—and yet, if I'm lucky, my hair will end up in the realm of "passable," not "perfect." This infuriates me. I am a beauty expert, damn it! Should I not be able to master these tricks and perform a perfect blowout on myself? Is it not my right? I may never have the answer. In the meantime, I comfort myself with the following tricks, which, though they may never be as good as Marcello's prowess, produce the next best (cheaper) thing.

THE TOOLS YOU WILL NEED

▶ Clips

▶ An ionic or ceramic blow-dryer

▶ A paddle brush

▶ Silicone serum and grooming cream

▶ A flatiron or curling iron

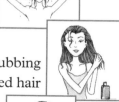

Step 1: Shampoo and condition with a sleek-ifying conditioner (look for ingredients like "silicone" on the back).

Step 2: Gently pat—don't rub—hair dry. Rubbing it will only annoy the cuticles, and annoyed hair cuticles = frizz.

Step 3: Rub a dime-sized (for short hair) or quarter-sized (for long hair) amount of silicone serum or heat-styling cream in your hands, then starting from hair ends, apply it, working your way up to the roots. Your ends should have the most product, your roots, the least.

Step 4: Using a paddle or boar-bristle (not round) brush, blow dry hair, piece by piece, when it's still damp (not wet, not too dry). You've surely heard the advice about drying your hair haphazardly 80% of the way and then blowing and brushing out the last 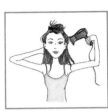 20%, but I find that, unless you are a true blow-dry expert 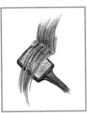 or have perfect hair to begin with, this often results in frizzy, fluffy hair. Instead, blot your hair with a towel (see above), then run a blow-dryer through your hair for about thirty seconds—just long enough to get rid of excess moisture. (Note: If achieving the perfect blowout is a daily routine for you, disregard the above and blow-dry your hair as much as possible before taking a brush to it, as brushing and blow-drying your hair from sopping wet to bone dry can take its toll.)

Step 5: Clip up the top of your hair (everything above your ears) and blow-dry starting in the back, working your way forward and up, doing the crown and pieces around your face last. (If they're too dry by the time you "arrive" there, wet your fingers and pull 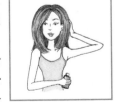 them through to redampen the strands.)

Step 6: Pull the brush tautly through your hair in small sections, aiming the blow-dryer nozzle down the hairshaft, so the airflow shoots down almost parallel to the strands. (This keeps you from roughing up the cuticle. Think about it; if you're aiming the nozzle toward your scalp, you're just going to end up with a million flyaways.)

Step 7: Apply finishing cream to your palms (good bets are Fekkai Glossing Cream or John Frieda Secret Weapon), rubbing hands together and then, beginning in the back and on the underside of hair—concentrating on ends and avoiding roots—running fingers through to smooth and hold the style.

Step 8: Go over any kinks with a flatiron (or, add texture with a curling iron, if you've suddenly developed a penchant for Kate Hudson–like hippie waves) and finish with a few spritzes of light-hold aerosol (read: not too wet) spray. (I love Bumble and bumble Does it All Spray and L'Oreal Elnett.)

BUT . . . IF YOU'RE IN A HURRY . . .

Sometimes you can't spare the necessary half-hour or forty-five minutes for the perfect blow-dry, and simply want to look semi-polished, fast. When that's the case, follow the steps above, but start with the pieces in the front of your head and surrounding your face. Spend a few minutes taking care to make the front pieces look smooth and polished, then quickly blow-dry (either with the paddle brush, or simply with your fingers if you're truly in a rush) the underneath and back, following with grooming cream and a few quick strokes of the flatiron on any wayward, cowlick-y pieces.

> **TIP:** *Experiencing flyaways, but stuck without hair cream? Use a dab of hand cream instead.*

∾ The List: Best Hairstyling Products

Ever wonder how your hair looks so damn good after you go to the salon, even if you *haven't* had a cut or highlights? Sure, blow-drying and styling technique have a little sump'in to do with it, but it's mostly thanks to the miracle of products. Whether you're looking to add volume, banish frizz, coax waves into curls, or simply look magazine-glossy, it's all about the stylers. Add these to your makeup cabinet, and you'll never have an "Oh-My-God-I'm-Just-Going-To-Shave-It-Off-And-End-It-All" bad-hair day again. Scout's honor.

Bumble and bumble Styling Spray: One of my all-time favorite products that works on all kinds of hair. Spray it on damp hair and then scrunch for curls, spray on damp hair before blow-drying for sleek locks with strong hold.

Fekkai Glossing Cream: With UVA/UVB sunscreen, this leave-in conditioner has a multitude of uses. Apply to damp hair before blow-drying or curling for heat protection and manageability, or to dry hair as a frizz-banisher and smoother. For soft, sweet-smelling waves, put a nickel-sized amount into damp hair, then pull into a loose bun or braid and secure for several hours before taking out.

Biosilk Silk Therapy: Excellent for very thick or coarse hair, with silk proteins to strengthen and protect while adding unbelievable smoothness and shine. Many of my friends with wiry, hard-to-comb-through hair that delights in doing *exactly* what you don't want it to swear by it. Just a tiny dab on wet hair before blow-drying works miracles.

Phytodefrisant: My favorite anti-frizz product; I won't even consider blow-drying without it. The botanical, chemical-free formula helps wavy hair achieve that coveted "stick straight" look without weighing it down into a greasy mess, and helps ease tight curls into loose ringlets.

Ouidad Climate Control Gel: Relaxes even the frizziest hair in the world into soft, well-defined curls. The more you use, the heavier and wetter the style, so if you like a natural look, just use a small dab.

Bumble and bumble Thickening Spray: I don't know what the hell they put in this stuff, but if it works even on my best friend, who has the flattest, most limp hair (that positively refuses to hold a style for even five minutes) in the world, then it'll work for you, too.

Aveda Shampure shampoo: Gentle enough to use daily, with a relaxing, orange-y scent and calming essences from flowers and plants. Whenever I get bored of my tricked-out shampoo of the moment, this is the wonderful old standby I always come back to.

TIP: *If you have curly hair and want to make it sleeker, use a straightening cream instead of a curling cream to help relax your strands.*

∾ Face Shapes and Haircuts

A good hairstylist will be able to disregard standard classifications about face shapes and haircuts to decide what kind of style will work for you based on several factors. "A person's height, weight, personality, and bone structure all influence what cut is right for them," says Edward Tricomi, co-owner of Warren-Tricomi salon in New York. For your own purposes, however (hey, knowledge is power, right?), here's a general guide.

If your face is ROUND

Although you might sometimes feel as if you have a pumpkin on your head, take heart—those rounded, babyish cheeks are going to serve you well in your old age, my dear. In the meantime, look for cuts with volume on top, very long, sideswept bangs (but never heavy, thick, straight-across ones!), or graduated layers. Avoid short, blunt cuts that will only serve as a picture-frame to your roundness.

Famous celebs: Julia Stiles, Kirsten Dunst, Kelly Osbourne, Drew Barrymore

If your face is OVAL

Consider yourself blessed. Chicks with oval-shaped faces can pull off just about every hairstyle under the sun. Not for nothing does almost every top model have an oval-shaped face. (Is this evolution, or just God being really biased and unfair? Who knows?) Garrison recommends a sexy shag with angled bangs.

Famous celebs: Natalie Portman, Sienna Miller, Kate Moss, Sharon Stone

If your face is HEART-SHAPED

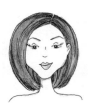

To minimize your cute chin, avoid too-short styles (which could make you look like a pixie—just add pointy ears!), and instead go for longer layers, a shoulder-length bob, or long-sideswept bangs.

Famous celebs: Reese Witherspoon, Jennifer Love Hewitt, Jennifer Aniston, Lisa Kudrow

If your face is SQUARE

Your wonderfully angular jaw gives you an edge in the bone-structure sweepstakes, but also means that you need to look for softening cuts to downplay it. Think either long and overly feminine, with angles past the chin, or short and textured. Avoid anything too geometric, like face-framing bangs or blunt-cut bobs.

Famous celebs: Gwyneth Paltrow, Demi Moore, Sandra Bullock, Jada Pinkett-Smith

If your face is LONG

Extremely long or extremely short cuts are often not the most flattering, as these can make your face appear even longer. Instead, look for ways to create the illusion of width, such as with bangs, a chin-length bob, or long layers. Avoid too much height at the crown when creating up-dos.

Famous celebs: Sarah Jessica Parker, Liv Tyler, Hilary Swank, Gabrielle Reece

∾ Your Hair Glossary

"A shag with long layers, fringe, and a few angles to bring out your cheekbones?" Um, yeah, whatever *that* means. So that you may never be stuck at the salon nodding in confusion again, Tricomi, Rivera, and Garrison explain a few basic hair-lingo definitions.

Angles

Frames that shape around the face

Crop

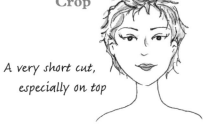

A very short cut, especially on top

Blunt

A cut that's all the same length: straight on the bottom with no layers

Feathered

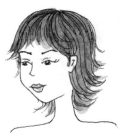

An angled, layered cut with wispy edges

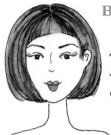

Bob

A cut, typically short, that's all one length

Long Layers

Different lengths cut into hair to create volume

Fringe

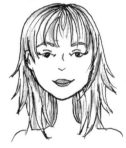

Bangs

Graduated Bob

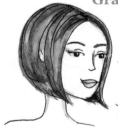

A cut that's short in back, with hair gradually longer in the front

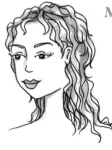

Mullet

Retarded haircut (Note: Well. There you have it. It's actually a cut that is short in front and long in the back.)

Pixie

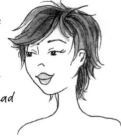

A soft and wispy cut
that's close to the head

Shag

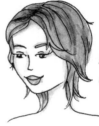

Highly layered haircut
of any length

Tunneling

Cutting out hair
underneath and inside

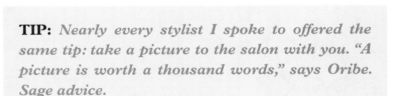

TIP: *Nearly every stylist I spoke to offered the same tip: take a picture to the salon with you. "A picture is worth a thousand words," says Oribe. Sage advice.*

∾ The Genius of Hair Powder

You're lazy. You're sleepy. You're already too late for work to shower. And you're in possession of fantastically (horrifically) dirty hair. What to do? Reach for hair powder. (Tada!) This stuff is miraculous. By sopping up the oil on your scalp and along your hair strands, your locks will have the appearance of being cleaner than they actually are . . . which is to say, probably not at all. It works particularly well if you'd like to throw your hair into a chic ponytail or bun—preferably one accessorized with a scarf or headband—but are worried that the general look you're giving off is "Dirty homeless hippie who has come into possession of a cute scarf or headband." Spray or sprinkle onto hair roots, then shake or brush it through. (Just make sure you're not wearing your favorite shirt while doing so.) Bumble and bumble makes a popular colored aerosol version; Klorane Extra Gentle Dry Shampoo Spray, retro drugstore brand Pssst! and Oscar Blandi Pronto Dry Shampoo are also good alternatives.

TIP: *Wash your hair as infrequently as you can get away with to avoid stressing and overdrying strands. When people start avoiding your cubicle at work and passing up empty adjoining seats on the subway, that's your cue to increase the frequency of washes.*

∾ The List: Hair Tools That Will Change Your Life

Just as Hollywood celebrities rely on an arsenal of stylists, makeup artists, and hair "geniuses" to help craft their look and create the illusion of being prettier, sexier, and smarter than us mere mortals (well, prettier, at least), a great hair day is not achieved on rainbows and prayers alone. Make friends with the right styling tool, and you, too, can reach the coveted paradise of Jennifer Anistonland.

Chi Ceramic Original Flatiron: No other iron does as good a job of heating up as quickly, cooling down as fast, and, of course, transforming frizzy, wavy hair into smooth, pin-straight tresses. It's expensive, but if you frequently battle your hair, the time and effort saved will be worth every penny. (Bonus: the ceramic plates mean the iron warms up evenly and makes it less likely to singe your hair. Regardless, always use heating tools with styling products specifically designed to protect your hair from damage.)

Solano Sapphire Flatiron: Heavier than the Chi, the Solano has the advantage (or disadvantange, depending on your point of view) of larger plates, which comes in handy when you need to straighten your hair very quickly, if you have very long hair, or if you have a lot of it. I have an unnatural attachment to my Solano—it is by far my personal favorite hairstyling tool. (Because I am lazy and it lets me do half the work for twice the results? Indeed.)

T3 Tourmaline Featherweight Professional Ionic Hair Dryer: Ionic hair dryers work with your hair (the ions in the dryer carry a negative charge, as opposed to the positively charged molecules in your strands) to cut drying time drastically. This beloved powerhouse takes it one step further with crushed tourmaline, the most potent ionic mineral in the world. Translation: hair that's so sleek (and dries so quickly), you could swear your stylist was right there in the bathroom with you. Unfortunately, it's not cheap. Like, at all. (Of course, it's not as expensive as the also amazing T3 Evolution, which is even *more* powerful and dries hair even *more* quickly—but costs enough to feed children in starving countries for the rest of their natural born lives. So, you choose.)

Mason Pearson Bristle and Nylon Brush: The Ferrari of hairbrushes. I don't normally advocate fibbing, but if you're, say, married and decide to buy this brush, allow me to make it easier for you: don't tell your husband how much it costs. Just lie. It will be better for everybody. The quality of the brush and bristles means that it not only lasts for years (and years . . . and years) but works to gently detangle hair, redistribute natural oils, stimulate the scalp to increase blood flow, and keep even fragile strands in great condition. The mere act of brushing your hair is actually harmful, so if your hair is even remotely fussy, pamper it with the best.

Just Like Grandma Used to Make— the Best Folk Remedies

For dry or brittle hair: Heat olive oil and massage into dry locks and scalp. Leave on for at least twenty minutes, then shampoo out.

For extra softness: Slather on Crisco or mayonnaise and eggs for softening, deep conditioning benefits.

When you're in a pinch and need hairspray or mousse: Use beer! According to Garrison, "Beer is the world's strongest-holding mousse. But beware, your hair will smell like a bar!"

How to: Curl Your Hair

A couple of years back, I was obsessed with the Olsen twins. No, not because I'm secretly some pervy old man who had the various "Days Until Mary-Kate and Ashley Turn Eighteen!" webpages bookmarked, but because I was in love with their loose, tousled waves and coveted the hair for myself. (This was before they started dressing like hobos. Ahh, the good old days.) Kate Hudson was also in possession of said miracle waves, and I'd flip through magazines, tearing out ads, photo shoots and paparazzi shots of the girls to paste on my wall at work for inspiration. I spent countless hours that year in front of my bathroom mirror (what's new?), trying to recreate the hair for myself. So, here you go—straight from my bathroom to yours.

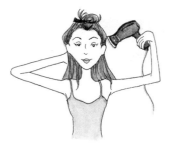

2. Clip hair up, then pull out large one-and-a-half-inch chunks.

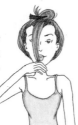

1. Apply a styling lotion or gel (my faves: Bumble and bumble Styling Spray and Phytodefrisant . . . what? They work!) to damp hair and then blow dry smooth, using the technique described above.

3. Use a wide-barreled curling iron.

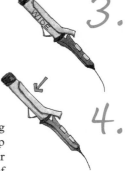

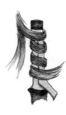

5. Hold the curling iron straight up and down, parallel to your head, and wrap sections of hair around the *outside* of the barrel for ten seconds, holding the bottom inch of your hair in your fingers.

4. Keep the curling iron clamped *shut.*

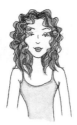

6. Continue until entire head is curled, with ends straight.

7. Tousle hair with fingers and pull a light styling cream through ends.

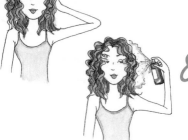

8. Finish with a spritz of hairspray.

∽ BEAUTY CONFIDENTIAL:
Hair Today, Gone Tomorrow

Despite being a "beauty expert"—or, perhaps, because of it—I've had numerous harrowing beauty experiences in my life, nearly all of them involving my hair. I'm going to admit it—I'm very, very vain about my locks. The older I get, the better I am at realizing that it's what's on the inside that counts, that having frizzy or dirty hair for an afternoon doesn't make me a bad person, that it *is* possible to still be attractive with air-dried hair (I think.) That being said, let's be real: beautiful hair just makes you feel better. Freshly washed tresses; a perfect blowout; glistening, shiny color—this is the stuff that beauty dreams are made of. So, when I have a new hair disaster, I take a deep breath, remind myself that it's only temporary, and then immediately set about trying to undo the damage. In a very zen-like, non-narcissistic kind of way, *of course.*

The first time I burned off a huge chunk of my hair, thereby rendering it mop-like for several months (oh, yes, there has been more than one time that this has happened), I was on a once-in-a-lifetime trip to Egypt for a cousin's wedding. We had a hairdresser come to our Cairo hotel room the afternoon of the wedding, armed with an arsenal of beauty tools. I decided that I would wear my hair down, visions of long, loose, soft ringlets dancing through my head. I sat patiently in the chair as the hairdresser worked silently, not bothering to look up from my magazine as he rolled locks this way and that with his hot iron. He finished, spritzed it with hair spray, and I floated downstairs to the ballroom, ready to pose for all the night's photos. When I look back at those pictures, it still brings a small, pathetic tear to my eye. I didn't know it then, but it was the end of a hair era.

Two days later, I arrived home to New York and washed my hair, ready to get back to work for the first time in over a week. As I rinsed out the shampoo, I suddenly realized that something was wrong. Wait a minute . . . was that . . . no . . . it couldn't be . . . but . . . yes . . . it was . . .

Clumps of hair. Dropping into the drain. *My* hair.

I quickly finished rinsing, slapped conditioner on it, and then stepped out of the shower in horror to survey the damage. My locks were—there's no other word for it—*fried.* The ends were broken off, curled up, and spiraling this way and that, floating inches away from my head as if I were channeling an electric current. You couldn't call the stuff on my head "hair." It was a Brillo pad.

So began my quest for the perfect intensive conditioner. My exhaustive search turned up several nourishing, revitalizing products, some of which even made the mop on my head *vaguely* resemble hair. No mean feat. And my newly learned, vast knowledge about different moisturizing hair treatments came in handy the following year when, having finally rehabilitated my hair and cut off all the dead bits, I burned it all off again. Sigh. My pain, your gain.

∾ The List: Best Intensive Conditioners

Even if you *haven't* fried your hair like an egg, intensive conditioners can do your tresses a world of good. Sun, heat, blow-drying, curling, flatironing, and brushing all take their toll on your locks, and—seeing as hair is basically just a collection of dead cells—most people's strands are desperately crying out for moisture. If your scalp is oily, apply only to the ends of hair; those with normal to dry scalps can get away with applying conditioner further up the hair shaft. Once a week (twice at most!) should do the trick.

Skin An Apothecary French Hair Paste: My numero uno, best-kept-secret hair conditioner—it practically demands to be applied by the handful, and it detangles like nobody's business. I've been addicted for years.

Aussie Three-Minute Miracle Deeeeep: A fruity, light conditioner that nevertheless works wonders on hair no matter what the condition, whether coarse, thin, frizzy, or limp. Equally effective as a daily conditioner and won't build up on the hair or drag it down. (Bonus: the drugstore price is very nice.)

Infusium: The best inexpensive leave-in conditioner around, and one of my all-time favorites. Use generously on wet or dry hair for added softness, moisture, and manageability.

Joico K-Pac Reconstructor: A banana-scented miracle in a bottle containing protein to help repair and rebuild even the most damaged, brittle hair. Ends breaking off into threes?

Bad bleach job? This is your product. Too much protein can actually be bad for the hair, however, so only use once a week, or even once every two weeks.

Kerastase Olèo-Relax: Just a dab goes a long way, leaving even fine hair soft, shiny, conditioned and in fantastic shape without weighing it down. Has a faint 1950's salon smell to it that some love, some hate.

L'Oreal Nature's Therapy Mega Moisture Hair Treatment: Excellent for coarse, severely damaged hair, with a mango scent and (by the by) an ingredient list almost identical to that of the popular conditioner Masquintense, by L'Oreal-owned Kèrastase. Perhaps a bit too heavy for fine or thin hair.

Terax Original Crema: We've already discussed the fabulosity of this particular conditioner—which works as both an intensive treatment and a daily nourisher—but it bears repeating. Use it. Love it.

Terax Original Lotion Life Drops: If you've pummeled your hair into oblivion through too much flatironing, blow-drying, bleaching, highlighting (you get the picture), apply a small amount of this powerhouse lotion to your wet hair after shampooing and conditioning. It's protein-based, so it will help rebuild and strengthen hair miraculously and quickly, but don't overuse.

∾ How To: Air Dry Your Wavy Hair So It Doesn't Look Like Frizzy, Fried Crap

If the world were solely comprised of models, Kate Hudson movie characters and chicks who'd undergone

Japanese thermal straightening, we would all step out of the shower, toss our tresses around, and, five minutes later, be blessed with perfectly straight, frizz-free, bouncy hair. Wouldn't that be nice? Can't you imagine it? No halo of damaged, bent strands around your crown; no splitting, crimped-out, waffle-like ends; no flat, lifeless locks; no cowlicks; no frizz. I say it again: *no frizz*. Sigh. Perhaps one day, my friends. Perhaps one day. In the meantime, the reality is this: unless you are one of God's genetically blessed, your hair probably does *not* look its best an hour after you wash it, especially if you're prone to hair twirling, especially if you never use product, especially if your hair has an evil mind of its own ("Hmm, she just got tossed in a pool right in front of the guy she likes. Wouldn't a cowlick and weird, asymmetrical flippy ends be an awesome thing to do right now?!"), and *especially* if you live in a "fun" climate zone like humid Florida (read: the 'fro-zone) or parched Arizona (read: hair like a limp noodle). Of course, you have to be a very committed, appearance-occupied gal to blow-dry and style your hair every . . . single . . . day, to say nothing of the havoc heat-styling wreaks on your locks anyway. So, what to do? Live a life of healthy-but-bad hair days, or fry the crap out of your strands for the sake of a pretty-but-secretly-mop-like-and-crying-out-for-moisture style? Fret not—there is a middle ground. If you learn how to airdry your waves properly (Yes! There *are* things you can do to make a visible difference), then you can alternate air drying it with blow drying it. Now, I'm not saying that your hair will look ready for *Glamour* magazine—but at least you won't look like you belong on the cover of *Poodle Weekly*, either.

1. Shampoo and condition hair, then squeeze out the excess moisture.
2. Comb hair, arranging the part where you'd like your hair to fall.
3. Apply several drops of leave-in conditioner or anti-frizz styling cream to towel-dried hair.
4. Spritz on styling lotion.
5. Scrunch hair with fingers and twirl into curls.
6. Once curls are arranged the way you like, hands off! (Touching will only result in the dreaded frizz.)

∽ Favorite Iconic Cuts

The Chanel Bob: In the roaring twenties, a generation of young girls rebelled against Victorian-era stuffiness by chopping off their hair to reject traditional notions of what it meant to be female. Elders were scandalized as girls cropped their hair close to their heads, wore pants and smoked like the boys. The precursor to today's rebellious teenage girls, who, instead of dressing like boys to piss off their parents, instead anger them by looking like porn stars. (Oops! Did I write that down? I only meant to think it.)

Veronica Lake: Notoriously shy, 40's film star Lake adopted this style as a way to hide behind her hair. The shiny, rolled wave covering one eye added allure and glamour—and proved millions of mothers wrong when they told their teenage daughters that hair in their faces looked messy.

Marilyn Monroe: On anybody else, short, white hair could appear almost dowdy, but on Marilyn, the softly rolled, platinum curls were sex itself. Her body and face may have had something to do with it, but, you know, the hair helped.

Farrah Fawcett: Over thirty years later, those famous flippy "wings" still evoke fun, sun, and 70s-style tackiness. Gorgeous on Farrah, but hard to pull off for us mere mortals.

The Rachel: When Chris McMillan cut Jennifer Aniston's thick hair into a long layered and angled shag during the second season of *Friends*, could anybody have predicted the insane reaction that followed? The cut (as you probably remember—you *so* ran to your local salon for "the Rachel," didn't you?) catapulted Aniston—and her hair—to megafame, and instantly turned McMillan into one of the hottest hairdressers in H-town.

Meg Ryan's Shag: Created by celebrity-stylist Sally Hershberger for Meg's 1995 movie *French Kiss*, this choppy, messy cut instantly became synonymous with Meg and her cheerful, girl-next-door persona. It carried her through for years and became something of a trademark, only failing her with that whole Russell Crowe/*Proof of Life* debacle. Goes to show that good hair can only get you so far, then— uh-oh!—morality takes over.

AND A FEW HAIRCUTS THAT WERE SO WRONG,
    THEY WERE RIGHT . . .

Scarlett Johansson: I can't picture any other sexy young actress with the *cojones* to chop her gorgeous tresses into a layered, razored mullet that wouldn't have looked out of place on a 70s truck driver . . . or Billy Ray Cyrus. But Scarlett went there—and frankly, I think she rocked it. After all, isn't beauty all about experimentation, anyway? What's a little mullet in the long-term glamour stakes?

Ali McGraw: Many loved this style, but I don't know if you can exactly call "long, straight, and parted down the middle like Wednesday Addams" a *style*. Perfect on Ali, lovely on gorgeous chicks, nine-times-out-of-ten unflattering for the rest of us. Still, completely emblematic of the "Eh, whatever, man. Hey, got a joint?" unfussiness of the 70s.

Sinead O'Connor: What could be more of a statement than just chopping it *all* off? Only to be attempted if you are insanely freaking gorgeous or Natalie Portman. (Or, in her case, both.)

TIP: *Starting to lose hair? Celebrity stylist Eliut Rivera recommends a mixture of carrot juice and caffeine applied to the scalp.*

∞ The Best Scalp Treatments

Scalps aren't sexy. They aren't cute. You can't, like, put makeup on them to highlight their inner beauty or anything. But they *are* insanely important to the health and beautiful appearance of your hair. After all, your hair is dead. But the stuff underneath your scalp? Totally alive. Keep your hair in great shape and increase the speed it grows at by massaging your scalp regularly to increase circulation and exfoliate follicle-clogging flakes. Once a month, massage a generous amount of scalp treatment—good ones to try include Philip B Rejuvenating Oil, JF Lazartigue Stimulactine 21, and Nioxin Recharging Complex—into your dry hair and scalp, then let sit for at least half an hour, if not longer, before shampooing out. I like to pull my hair into a bun and use a hairdryer while the product is in my hair, to help open up the shaft and let the ingredients penetrate deeper. You'll notice less scalp buildup and shinier, better-conditioned hair almost immediately.

> **TIP:** *Hair growing slowly? Try nail-and-hair growth vitamins containing keratin, such as Appearex, which you can find at the drugstore and which can make a dramatic difference.*

CHAPTER TWO PRODUCT PRICE GUIDE

$: less than $10
$$: between $10 and $24
$$$: between $25 and $49
$$$$: between $50 and $100
$$$$$: more than $100

Products

Flawless by Danilo, $$$, *ultimatelooks.com*
Ken Paves, $$$$, *hairuwear.com*
Frederic Fekkai Glossing Cream, $$, *sephora.com*
John Frieda Secret Weapon, $, drugstores
Bumble and bumble Does It All Styling Spray, $$,
    bumbleandbumble.com for locations
L'Oreal Elnett hairspray, $$, *zitomer.com*
Bumble and bumble Styling Spray, $$, *bumbleandbumble.com*
    for locations
Biosilk Silk Therapy, $$, *farouk.com* for locations
Phytodefrisant, $$$, *phyto-usa.com* for locations
Ouidad Climate Control Gel, $$, *ouidad.com*
Bumble and bumble Thickening Spray, $$,
    bumbleandbumble.com for locations
Aveda Shampure Shampoo, $$$, *aveda.com*
Bumble and bumble Hair Powder, $$,
    bumbleandbumble.com for locations
Klorane Extra Gentle Dry Shampoo Spray, $$,
    metrobeauty.com

Pssst! Dry Powder Spray, $$, drugstores

Oscar Blandi Pronto Dry Shampoo, $$, *oscarblandi.com*

Chi Ceramic Original Flatiron, $$$$$, *farouk.com* for locations

Solano Sapphire Flatiron, $$$$, *folica.com*

T3 Tourmaline Featherweight Professional Ionic Hair Dryer, $$$$$, *nordstrom.com*

T3 Tourmaline Evolution Hair Dryer, $$$$$, *nordstrom.com*

Mason Pearson Bristle and Nylon Brush, $$$$, *zitomer.com*

Skin An Apothecary French Hair Paste, $$, *skinanapothecary.com*

Aussie Three-Minute Miracle Deeeeep, $, drugstores

Infusium, $, drugstores

Joico K-Pac Reconstructor, $$, *joico.com* for locations

Kerastase Olèo-Relax, $$$, *kerastase.com* for locations

L'Oreal Nature's Therapy Mega Moisture Hair Treatment, $, drugstores

Terax Original Crema, $$, *sephora.com*

Terax Original Lotion Life Drops, $$, *sephora.com*

Philip B Rejuvenating Oil, $$$, *philipb.com*

JF Lazartigue Stimulactine 21, $$$$, *jflazartigue.com*

Nioxin Recharging Complex, $$, *nioxin.com* for locations

Appearex, $, drugstores

Salons and Experts

Louis Licari salon, 693 Fifth Avenue, New York, NY:
212–758–2090

Mark Garrison salon, 108 East 60th Street, New York, NY:
212–400–8000

Oribe salon, 1627 Euclid Avenue, Miami Beach, FL:
305–538–8006

Ken Paves salon, 409 North Robertson Boulevard, Los Angeles,
CA: 310–499–7122

Warren-Tricomi salon, 16 West 57th Street, New York, NY:
212–262–8899

Salon Eliut Rivera, 762 Madison Avenue, New York, NY:
212–472–3440

Three

Hair Color

*Blondes don't necessarily have more fun, but
salons sure as hell want you to think they do
(Or: How a TV show changed my life)*

I was fourteen years old when I lost my hair color virginity.
It was 1994 and *My So-Called Life*, the critically acclaimed
but viewer-ignored TV show starring Claire Danes as Angela
Chase, was all the rage among my friends in Alpharetta, Georgia. We swooned over Jordan Catalano, suffered through Angela's indignities as though they were
our own, and marveled over how
Claire Danes just *so* got it and was
the coolest thing ever. I coveted her
life, geeky next-door neighbor Brian
Krakow and all. Mostly, though, I
coveted her aubergine-red hair. My
own hair had been a light, sunny

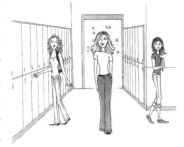

shade of beachy blond my entire childhood, but suddenly took
a turn for the dishwater brown *juuuust* when I hit those oh-so-

crucial middle-school years. (Thanks, God! Fun joke!) Brown hair is often glamorous, mysterious, sexy. My hair was none of these things. It was flat. It was faded. At times, in the wrong light, it almost looked dark gray. In short, it was the kind of color that begged—nay, demanded!—to be dyed.

I needed a few weeks to gather up the courage to dye it, terrified that my parents would disown me if I suddenly turned up one day with Manic Panic locks. (Isn't it kind of quaint to look back and remember the innocuous things you thought of as "bad behavior" in your early teens?) I finally mustered the will to talk to my mother about it as we drove though town one day, telling her, "Mom, we need to talk." When I confessed that I was planning on dying my hair red like Claire Danes's that weekend, she seemed relieved as if thinking, "Oh, is *that* all?" We then plotted about how to tell my father—although all of the worrying was for naught, since his only comment after the at-home dye job was, "Did you get a haircut?" Men.

When I turned up at school the day after going red, I felt like a rock star. (It was, in fact, destined to be one of many rock-star hair experiences in my life, such as the time I showed up at the office with ten inches of brand-new Barbie-like hair extensions, or the day I left work for four hours as a long-haired blonde and returned with short, nearly-black locks.) Friends stopped me at my locker, trailing wisps of my hair through their fingers and marveling at the new color. Classmates stared after me as I walked down the hallway or entered rooms, then did double-takes as they realized who I was, squealing, "Oh my *God*! Your hair looks so *good*!" I even merited a glance or two from the popular girls, who—in retrospect—were probably just looking behind me in the cafeteria to see where their football player boyfriends were. At the time, however, I was convinced that they were eyeballing me approvingly, thinking, "That Nadine sure does have great hair." (Cut me some slack—I *was* only fourteen.)

Regardless, it was my first experience with the transformative power of hair color. I was, understandably, hooked.

The color only lasted a few weeks before it became dull and lifeless, with no hint of the vibrance I'd initially enjoyed. After the thrill of first dye, my hair suddenly looked boring! What was I to do? Well, obviously, dye it again. I decided not to use the exact same color, going instead a slightly lighter, more realistic shade of red that is *occasionally* found in nature. More compliments at school. More obliviousness from Dad. More being convinced that I was moving closer and closer to popular. More thrills upon realizing the power of hair.

I went lighter. And then lighter still. I fled Georgia to attend boarding school in California for my senior year of high school—sounds so mysterious, no?—and kept on dying. By the time I returned to Alpharetta for a Spring Break visit to my old high school, I was a full-fledged blonde. The reaction was astounding. Compounded with the fact that I'd lost ten pounds and cut my hair into a neat bob, my newly blond locks set the hallways abuzz, and this time, it *wasn't* just my imagination. (Several years later, in college, a visiting high-school friend regaled me with tales of friends, acquaintances, and strangers alike discussing my *She's All That* transformation the day I returned. I took particular joy in hearing that a boy who had teased me mercilessly in middle school had declared I suddenly looked "really hot.")

What I love about hair color is the ability to completely transform yourself depending on what shade you're currently rocking. As a redhead, men three times my age had no problem stopping me on the street and telling me how sexy it was. (That's very traumatic when you're fifteen, by the way. Just, ew.) When I'm a blonde, I turn heads as I enter bars and get wolf whistles from men on streets. Lest I get too cocky and think it has anything to do with how I actually *look*, however, I have my brunette experiences to burst my bubble: with dark hair—even in various rich, chocolately, mahogany incarnations—it's as if I'm invisible. No free drinks at bars. No wolf whistles. Only people who I've known for years suddenly asking, "Hey, are you, like, half-Asian?" (Important note: I'm not saying that blondes are inherently sexier or more noticeable than brunettes. Some of the sexiest women in the world are brunettes, *obviously*. I just have no hope of, say, winning the Miss Universe pageant as a brunette. Well, not as a blonde, either, but that has more to do with the fact that I'm not five-ten with thighs like an eleven-year-old . . . anyhow. Moving on.)

Less than 20% of American women are natural blondes, but you wouldn't know that by flipping through a magazine or walking around on the street. My theory? It's because salons love doling out the blond: it requires tons of upkeep to keep roots from growing in and highlights are enormously expensive. Whether you're a blonde, brunette, redhead or, hell, a Smurf, here's the rundown on everything hair-color-related.

❧ Just the Facts, Please

According to Clairol:

- 39% of American women who color their hair go blond
- 37% of American women who color their hair go brunette
- 18% of American women who color their hair go redhead
- Only 19% of people are naturally blond
- 55 million American women dye their hair, with 36 million women doing it at home.
- 49% of first-time hairdye users are under the age of 17

❧ Expert Tip

LOUISE GALVIN'S SALON LINGO

Have you ever heard stylists talk about the difference between ashy and buttery color and thought: "Whaaa?" With all the words they're throwing around—not to mention the difference between my "two inches" and those of most stylists—it's a miracle you leave the salon looking even remotely as you'd hoped. I spoke with London-based celebrity colorist Louise Galvin for a cheat sheet—so you'll know *exactly* what your colorist means when she says she's taking you "cool blond with buttery lowlights."

Ashy: A shade that, on brunettes, includes no red; on blondes, is creamy without any gold.

Buttery: A golden, sun-kissed shade. Think Kate Hudson.

Golden: A sun-kissed effect, similar to buttery.

Warm: A shade that appears chestnut-toned on brunettes; golden and buttery on blondes; a golden color on redheads.

Cool: A shade that appears creamy and white-ish, without golden tones, on blondes; ashy with no red on brunettes; bluish, not golden, on redheads.

Balayage: Method of applying highlights and lowlights without foils, by painting directly onto hair.

Highlights: Color painted on the hair to add light; only applied in certain places, not on the whole head; usually most common on the top of head and around the face.

Lowlights: Darker color painted on the hair to add depth and color; usually applied in conjunction with highlights.

Bleach lights: The stripping of the natural pigment down to a very light blond.

Base color: The all-over color of your hair, in contrast to the highlights or lowlights applied (i.e.: a brown base with blond highlights).

Single-Process: Coloring the entire head and/or roots.

Double-Process: Coloring the entire head and/or roots, then adding highlights on top.

FACT: *In the years since the Miss America pageant began in 1921, 70% of the winners have been brunettes. (Only 24% have been blondes, and 6% have been redheads.)*

∾ How To: Dye Your Hair At Home

If you've ever watched a hair-color professional at work, it looks so easy. All you do is slop the color on, make sure it's evenly distributed, wait approximately twenty minutes, and voila! Instant gorgeous color. Must be easy to replicate at home, right? Wrong, of course. The color goes all over the bathroom, your ears and forehead end up purple for two days, somehow you miss several patches on the sides and in the back, and the color never looks as good as it does on the box. And that's when you're lucky, and don't end up with, say, orange locks. What to do? Try these steps to brilliant at-home color (your friends will never know you did it yourself):

1. What kind of commitment are you looking for? A temporary tint? Color just to cover up some grays? A drastic color change? Subtle highlights? Highlights add texture and color to your hair, but are nearly impossible to do yourself properly. (Seriously. Just trust me on this one.) Semipermanent stains wash out after about 6–12 shampoos, but because no ammonia or peroxide is used, you can only darken your hair, not lighten it. Demi-permanent color is similar, but includes a small level of peroxide, so won't wash out for 24–26 shampoos and will produce a more noticeable color change. Finally, permanent color uses both ammonia and peroxide and can't be washed out. Not good for commitment-phobes.

2. Which shade? If you have a warm complexion and natural hair color, choose a new shade in the same family; ditto for cool. Warm-toned people tend to have reddish/

golden tones in their complexions and hair, whereas cool-toned people have bluish tints without any gold. Try avoiding shades from the contrasting color family; if you're cool, your options range from platinum to black; if you're warm, pick a color between strawberry blond to dark auburn. Regardless of your color choice, never go more than three shades lighter or darker at home; anything more drastic is a recipe for disaster and should be done at a salon. The colors on the box can be misleading, so think of it as a guide rather than fact, and realize that your end result will probably be a few shades darker (if you're trying to go light), or lighter (if you're going darker).

3. Even after you have the color narrowed down, it can be difficult to choose between the seemingly millions of different brands. If you have a friend who has successfully dyed her hair (note the word "successfully"), ask what brand she used. Otherwise, make sure to read the boxes, to avoid the easy mistake of buying a line for ethnic hair when you're naturally blond, or, say, permanent color when all you want is a tint that will shampoo out.

4. I know you're eager to get started, but take the time to do an allergy and strand test to ensure you won't get a rash and the color is right. The allergy test should be done at least two days before you dye to give it time to react. After mixing together the dye ingredients, smear a tiny dab on the inside of your elbow (one of the most sensitive parts of your skin) and leave it on for twenty-four hours. If nothing happens, you're good to go. The strand test can be done right

before you dye your hair: take a small amount of the dye and apply it with a gloved hand to a piece of hair on the underside of your head and follow dying instructions on the box.

5. Make sure everything is all ready to go when you dye; fumbling around for tools and directions is a surefire way to mess up. You'll need:

     a. Rubber gloves.
     b. Comb.
     c. Old clothes (cover up as much of your skin as possible with a ratty shirt and sweatpants you don't mind getting dyed).
     d. Towel/dishcloth (that you can throw out when you're done) to wipe off excess dye.
     e. Large plastic bag and hair clip.
     f. Timer.
     g. The directions: Read them thoroughly before you start so you know exactly what to do.

6. Follow the instructions exactly as written. You'll probably need to mix/shake some bottles together to start.

     a. After mixing, work the dye from the roots out. The hair should be completely and evenly soaked in color.
     b. Use a comb to help spread the color through your hair.
     c. Put the plastic bag over your hair, twisting it tightly, then secure it with a hair clip.
     d. Set the timer for the exact amount of time you

need. Do NOT leave it in longer! If you want stronger results, then use a hairdryer over the plastic bag.

e. After the timer goes off, remove the bag and take a shower. Use the special conditioner that comes with the kit—this is my favorite part of the entire at-home-hair-dying experience!

7. Remember that damaged hair accepts color more quickly than undamaged hair, so you may end up with a more streaky look than you intended. Most products allow you to reuse the dye for spot treatment, but others only last for around a half hour. Be sure which one you pick!

8. Invest in a good shampoo/conditioner set specifically made for colored hair. Most companies that make hair dyes that will also have a shampoo/conditioner line to make the color last. Roots will have to be touched up every 4–6 weeks, and instructions on how to do this are also included in the box.

TIP: *After coloring hair, don't wash it for a couple of days, to ensure that you don't shampoo away any of the color. As time goes by, your color will fade, so keep it vibrant with color-enhancing shampoos and conditioners. My favorite lines for color-treated hair are Kerastase and L'Oreal Professionnel Serie Expert, but John Frieda, Pantene, and ARTec also make stellar products specifically for blondes, brunettes, and redheads.*

∾ My Favorite Haircolor Style Icons

BLONDES

Grace Kelly: The ultimate cool blonde, and far and away my greatest personal style icon, Grace Kelly is the epitome of class and, well, grace. Even years before her royal wedding, Grace carried herself with the style and air of a princess. Her blond waves were always perfectly in place, her lipstick never smudged, her makeup beautiful without a hint of ostentation. If you looked carefully, her eyes belied something deeper and more dangerous burning within, but on the outside, Grace was as cool as a cucumber—and that's just the way I like her. When I'm getting ready for fancy events such as weddings and black-tie balls, Grace is the one I channel.

Catherine Deneuve: With the sunny good looks of a California girl mixed with heavy-lidded eyes and a sense of Parisian mystery, Catherine Deneuve is the perfect Franco-American combination that comes along once in a generation. (She is also, in my mind, the exact opposite of France's current poster child, *Amelie*'s Audrey Tautou, who looks Gallic to a T, but has that unique, childlike American whimsy that one finds so often on the West Coast.)

Gwyneth Paltrow: Sure, Gwyneth is Grace Kelly's heir apparent, but what is it really about her that holds such a fascination? Her teeth are sort of crooked, her nose is a little wider than is normal for a glamorous Hollywood star, and she looks like an albino without makeup. (Hey! Just like me!) I think it's two things: 1. She carries herself like a goddess. Treat yourself right, and others will follow suit. 2. She has really, *really* good hair. It's thick, it's (usually) long and it's the perfect color of blond that normally exists only in the nursery. (*Never* underestimate the power of blond.)

REDHEADS

Lucille Ball: The most famous redhead of them all, Lucy perfectly embodies several of the characteristic redhead traits—she was fiery and fun, passionate and playful, and never backed down from a confrontation. A true original, Lucy was a trailblazer in Hollywood, becoming the first woman head of a production studio, something practically unheard of in the male-dominated early 60s. Lucille was actually a natural blonde—it wasn't until she dyed her hair red that she began to make a name for herself.

Julia Roberts: Platinum, dark, brown, blond—Julia's hair has been through every shade. But the color that she'll forever be associated with is red. No other star of our generation has even come close to Julia's megawatt fame, glow, and charisma. Lest you think her power is only in her blinding smile, remember the furor that was caused when she chopped off her mane and dyed it blond for *Hook*? Or covered up her hair altogether for *Mary Reilly*? Exactly. Julia's best roles (*Pretty Woman, Steel Magnolias, My Best Friend's Wedding*) have all showcased her with those wild, curly red locks—just the way we like it.

Rita Hayworth: Perhaps the sultriest star ever to grace the big screen, Rita Hayworth's sexuality held equal parts of joy and sadness. In that famous scene from *Gilda*, when

Rita first appears on screen by flipping her hair and purring, "Me?" she became the most famous actress in the world and the war pinup for a generation. It was a distinction that would forever haunt her. Her most famous quote is heartbreaking—"Every man I knew went to bed with Gilda and woke up with me." Half Spanish, Rita had naturally dark hair, although, like Lucy, it was with the red that she transformed into a star.

BRUNETTES

Elizabeth Taylor: The epitome of the sultry, sexy brunette, La Liz was truly sex on heels, able to reduce a man to rubble or make him feel as powerful as a god with only one glance of those violet eyes. Her sex-goddess status hinted at a vulnerability that she only showed to her paramours in the bedroom—probably after a seriously wild night.

Audrey Hepburn: Has there ever been a more refined celebrity? Audrey glided through the world with dignity and ease, setting herself apart from everybody she encountered, as if an ethereal angel. Gamine and elfin, Audrey's cool charms were both detached and passionate at the same time. Elegance personified.

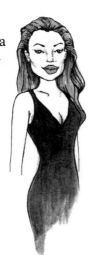

Angelina Jolie: Love her or hate her, Angelina is the modern Liz Taylor, burning her way through relationships and making an indelible mark on the world. And those lips! That tumbling mane! Those eyes! So feminine . . . yet so tough and almost masculine at the same time. Not for nothing does she seem to be at the top of every straight female's "If you had to, who would you do?" list. Yet, when Angie dyes her hair blond, her power mysteriously diminishes.

Tip: *Hair color can fade in the sun, so make sure you apply UV protective gel, spray, or cream before heading to the beach or a ball game—especially if you've dyed it recently.*

CHAPTER THREE PRODUCT PRICE GUIDE

$: less than $10
$$: between $10 and $24
$$$: between $25 and $49
$$$$: between $50 and $100
$$$$$: more than $100

Products

Kerastase, $$$, *kerastase.com* for locations
L'Oreal Professionnel Serie Expert, $$,
    us.lorealprofessionnel.com for locations
John Frieda, $, drugstores
Pantene, $, drugstores
ARTec, $$$, *us.lorealprofessionnel.com* for locations

Salons and Experts

Louise Galvin at Daniel Galvin Salon, 58–60 George Street,
    London, England: 44 (0)20 7486 9661

Four

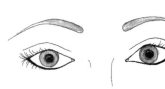

Eyes

*Making the most of
your sexiest feature*

When I was fifteen, I had a French exchange student visit me in Atlanta. We hit it off (or rather, I thought she was the coolest thing *ever* and she deigned to tolerate me) and so I went to visit her the following summer in St. Paul Trois-Châteaux, a small town in the south of France. I spent all of August there, which happened to include my sixteenth birthday—one of the best months of my entire life, even thus far. E. was a year older, athletic, tan, and blonde, with blue eyes, super white teeth, and dimples. Needless to say, all the boys loved her. (And me? Awkward, shy, hopeful, and just all-around embarrassing. Looking back on it makes me laugh, in a sort of happy, "Thank God that poor girl grew up" kind of way.) We took a week-long trip down to the French Riviera to visit her father, and spent our evenings walking on the beach with older French boys, drinking wine, and listening to French rap (Doc Gyneco, *tu me manques!*). Everything about E. oozed easy confidence, from her habit of casually flipping her hair, to the way she carefully doled out attention to the boys (a cutting roll of the eyes here, a playful slap and girlish giggle there). The thing that most impressed me, however, was E.'s eyeliner trick: lining her inner rims all the way around—on top and bottom—with a sharpened jet-black pencil. The effect was perhaps too harsh for her Nordic features (she looked completely different from all the other French girls, with their sultry Lou Doillon eyes, pouty lips, and olive skin), but it would transform her face, giving her eyes a fierce, leonine quality. It took months to master (my own liner would always smudge or somehow migrate to the inner corners of my eye, collecting at my tear ducts in masses of sticky black goop), but after I left France, it became one of my standard evening makeup maneuvers, and my finishing touch to this day. It was years before I learned that this trick wasn't unique to the fabulous E., but it still feels special to me. When I look in the mirror at the lined eyes staring back at me, I remember being an eager fifteen-year-old and hoping that I, too, could have some of E.'s stardust rub off on me. I remember when every precious evening held so much anticipation and promise, and those last moments of looking in the bathroom mirror at her villa before setting off on the night's adventures were both terrifying and thrilling. And, somehow, eye makeup seemed to be the crux of it all.

I still find myself reaching for the eyeliner pencil on special nights out, or pulling out the ol' smokey eye when I need a bit of extra sex kitten, but I've learned that more does *not* always equal better. Nothing is sexier than a sultry, shadowed eye, but the "I Slept in My Makeup Last Night" look? Unflattering, to say the least.

It's tempting to go one of two routes when wearing eyeshadow: no effort whatsoever or hooker. (Oh, you know exactly what I mean. Either it's a smudge of taupe-colored shadow that barely does anything for you, or it's ten pounds of grayish-black shadow that migrates onto your cheeks ten minutes after you apply it.) Believe it or not, eyeshadow isn't that difficult to apply. And, in my opinion, it's one of the cosmetics with the biggest payoff—even a tiny bit of the right shade will enhance your eye color, brighten your complexion, and polish your look. It amazes me how many of my friends don't know how to apply it properly, however, staring helplessly at their expensive eyeshadow compacts and asking me, "Well, where do I put *this* color? And *this* one?" Over the years, I've become the go-to gal for my friends on nights when they want to look their best, and their biggest wonder is never foundation or blush or bronzer or lipstick but always (always) eyeshadow: "How do you make my eyes look like that?? Show me!" As with everything, it takes a little trial and effort, so set aside some time one evening to play around and have fun. After all, that's what makeup should be about!

> *Pretty is something you're born with. But beautiful, that's an equal opportunity adjective.*
>
> *Anonymous*

∾ The Biggest Eyeshadow Mistakes

We've just mentioned two of the biggest eyeshadow errors: being terrified of wearing too much shadow, and so therefore wearing practically nothing and not enhancing your eyes (this may not seem like a makeup "crime" to some, but if you're going to make the effort, you might as well do it right, no?), or applying way, way, *way* too much. There is a middle ground, however, and its name is moderation. I like to apply eyeshadow with my fingers, so I can control the level of shadow and blend it easily into skin. If you use your fingers instead of a brush, make sure your hands are clean, otherwise the oils on your fingers will build up on the shadow over time and cause a film. (Eyeshadows will normally keep for about a year.)

⌒ If You Want a Casual Look

Start with a neutral eyeshadow color that's a few shades darker than your own skin tone. Using your fingers or an eyeshadow brush, apply the color on your lid, extending up to your browbone. Layer a slightly darker color, such as a taupe, light brown or light gray, either following the natural line made by your eyelid crease, so that you have a bit of the lighter shadow peeking out on your eyelid and brow bone, or apply the darker shadow on just your eyelid to frame your eyes. Finish with a few swipes of mascara, no eyeliner necessary.

⌒ If You Want a Daytime Look (i.e., for the Office or a Lunch Date) That's Pretty but Not Too Dramatic

The application method will be the same as above, but you simply need to apply eyeliner and a few extra coats of mascara. If you're daring or start to get bored by the same daily look, use a darker color along the crease of your eyes, or try applying a pale wash of a pretty color (such as violet, forest green, or powder blue) on your lids.

∾ If You Want a Sexy Nighttime Look

Two options: start with either a shimmery, champagne-colored shadow or a bronze-colored one and apply all over lids and extending up to just below the brow-bone. Apply a dark shadow (try rusty brown, deep plum, navy blue, gray, or emerald green) along the crease, following the natural curve of the eye, then blend well. Apply black, navy, or brown eyeliner (on both top and bottom, if you're feeling adventurous!), then use an eyelash curler and primer before several swipes of mascara. Or see below for instructions on the perfect smoky eye (my favorite!)

∾ How To: Create the Perfect (Not Too Tara Reid!) Smoky Eye

Not for nothing does almost every actress who walks the red carpet have a perfectly smudged, shadowed look. The dark shadow makes eyes pop and adds instant drama and glamour. If you're too heavy-handed, however, you'll look a mess—

probably a cross between Courtney Love and Tara Reid. (Hardly the desired effect.) The trick? Blend, blend, blend.

Step 1: Start with a clean, oil-free eye area (wash your face beforehand) and apply an eyeshadow primer (or a light dusting of translucent powder, in a pinch) to keep the area matte and help shadow stay longer.

Step 2: Pick an eyeliner (black, brown, gray, blue, purple . . . any color will do!) and apply it to your top lashes, keeping the line as close to the lash as possible. Use a Q-Tip to soften and smudge the line slightly, then repeat, applying and smudging again. (Optional: apply liner to the bottom of your eyes for a super-dramatic look. Keep the line as thin as possible and smudge gently, using an eyeliner brush or Q-tip to gently press on a tiny bit of translucent powder or eyeshadow in the same shade as the liner to set it.)

Step 3: Apply a light color over the entire area, from lids to browbone. Good options include champagne, pearl, and taupe-colored shadow.

Step 4: Follow with a dark color—go for black or gray for a traditional look, or try jewel-toned purple, blue, or green for a more modern smoky eye—applying it starting from your lash-line, and blending with an eyeshadow brush (it's best not to use fingers for a smoky eye, as the brush will deposit more pigment) all the way up to your eye crease. Blend well, making sure the dark shadow stays symmetrically within the contours of your outer eye (no dark smudges out near your temple!) and don't migrate above your crease. (Note: If you have eyes without much depth, such as typically Asian eyes, extend the dark shadow a tiny bit over the crease to create the illusion of a hollow.)

Step 5: Finish with several coats of volumizing or lengthening mascara (use a lash curler followed by eyelash primer, if you dare!).

TIP: *Celebrity makeup artist Nick Barose advises using a waterproof liner when creating a smoky eye, applying it both to the upper lash line and inside the lower lash line, and then blinking several times to gently smudge.*

∾ Picking an Eyeliner

Whether you have albino eyes like me or a naturally defined look (you lucky dog), eyeliner will give you that *yowza* factor that so often comes in handy (dates, weddings, Halloween parties where you're dressed as an angel or pirate or flower . . . I'm sorry, a *sexy* angel or pirate or flower). If you're unsure of your eyeliner abilities, pick a soft pencil that smudges easily (Stila Kajal liner is a great option). The standard eyeliner pencil tends to be a bit harder, and is better used when you're sure your hand won't be shaking all over the place. Try steadying your arm on your bathroom counter, or resting your wrist on your chin as you apply. Once you've mastered the art of lining, graduate to a liquid liner for night and more formal events; it'll give you that sexy, Liz Taylor cat-eye thing.

▸ Start in the inner corner of your eye and extend out.

▸ Apply a very thin line near your inner corner, making it thicker as you approach the outer edge of your eye.

▸ For extra drama, flick the line up very slightly at the outer corners.

▸ Apply liner as close as possible to your lash line.

▸ If you like the look of liner on both the top and the bottom (beware, this look smudges easily and can result in raccoon eyes), place just a few drops in between the lash line and then use an eyeliner brush or Q-tip to very lightly blend outward.

▸ To help liner stay put, dip an eyeliner brush in either translucent powder or eyeshadow that's the same color as your liner and press it on top of the lash line to "set."

∾ Beauty Myth: Never Wear Eyeshadow the Same Color As Your Eyes

This so-called rule drives me crazy. I'm supposed to discount an entire range of colors—Navy! Aqua! Cerulean!—just because my eyes have a hint of blue in them? No, no, no. Sure, if your eyes are baby blue, maybe you shouldn't walk around wearing turquoise shadow—but probably neither should anybody else (unless you're a so-called hipster or on your way to an 80s party, of course). Here's a cheat sheet to surprisingly great eye color/shadow color combinations.

If you have blue eyes: All you need is bronze. Mix it up with dark gray and baby blue.

If you have green eyes: Plum and violet will look phenomenal (just make sure they're not too pinky or reddish if you have a ruddy complexion), as well as very dark, dusky green.

If you have brown eyes: Go for vibrant colors like blues and greens, or highlighting champagnes and pale whites.

If you have hazel eyes: Neutral mushroom or taupe-colored shades contrasted with medium-hued greens or blues (depending on which way you want to take your eyes) will look divine.

Note: I'm willing to be corrected on this, but in my experience, maroon, rust, or bronze shadow makes *everybody* look sexier and enhances their eyes. Think about it: the color basically mimics a tan, so it warms up your face and makes any eye color pop.

TIP: *Want to wear a certain crazy eyeshadow color, but afraid of looking like a circus performer? Use your normal eyeshadow but add a pop of color as an eyeliner, or apply the vibrant shade over your regular eyeshadow, either in the crease or on the lid, for just a hint of color.*

∾ Eyebrows

When I got all angsty at the beginning of high school, I decided a good way to deal with it would be to take it out on my eyebrows. (I also wrote terrible poetry, wore boys' clothes, listened to grunge, and pierced my ears myself—it was the early 90s, what do you want from me?—but that's another story for another time.) I've never had heavy brows, or particularly dark hair, but my brows were nonetheless a completely misshapen mess and desperately needed a shape—any shape. Except for the shape I went with. Which was completely off. Yes, in the wake of the Kate Moss/waif model craze and 80s backlash, no brows at all suddenly seemed like my answer. And so I plucked and plucked and plucked some more, late into the night, until I was left with two limp, sad little arches over my eyes. My mother was less horrified, more simply baffled. ("But, but . . . *why?*") Poor little misguided teenager that I was, I actually thought that it was a good look for me. A year later, on a whim, I started growing my brows out, suddenly having decided that the Brooke Shields look *was* cool again. (For this, I blame Madonna. I don't know why . . . but I just do.) It wasn't until I read some magazine article, probably in *InStyle*, my obsession at the time, about how to tend to your brows that I learned how to properly pluck them. (That was the end of my "tadpole" phase, thank God.)

It's pretty amazing that getting rid of just a few strays on your face can make such a huge difference, but it does. Not only is it cleaner-looking, but it also opens up the area around your eye, making you look younger and fresher and serving as an instant eyelift. (Sounds stupid, but it's true.) If you've never had your eyes professionally groomed before, I strongly recommend going to a salon and having them done, then performing the upkeep yourself. Once a professional assesses what shape will be best for your eyes and face, you can then spend one or two minutes every week maintaining it by removing errant hairs.

∾ How To: Tweeze Your Brows

Step 1: Place a magnifying mirror next to a window to maximize the light and see all the tiny hairs.

Step 2: Look at the natural curve of your brow; you're going to want to work with it, not alter it dramatically. Find where your arch should be by holding the base of a pencil (yes, this old-school trick still works!) parallel against the tip your nose, and then turning it so that the pencil is on top of your iris. The tip of the pencil will hit a spot on your brow; that's the area where your arch should be.

Step 3: Pluck only one hair at a time, starting at the arch area and working outward toward your temples. Tweeze the hair under your brow only. Slant-tip tweezers work best; for an easier, less painful pluck, pull out the hair parallel to your skin, rather than yanking it out perpendicularly.

Step 4: Once you've finished cleaning up the arch area (taking care not to shorten the length of your brows; they should extend at least beyond the corner of your eyes), remove stray hairs from in between your brows, and the area above the inner corner of your eyes. Hold the pencil parallel to the side of your nose; it'll hit the brow right at the place where it should start.

Step 5: After tweezing, groom your brows with eyebrow gel or an old, washed mascara wand, brushing them up so you can see if there are any long hairs that need to be trimmed. If necessary, use small scissors to trim the inner corners of your brows, above the nose and inner corner of the eyes. Don't overtrim!

Step 6: Apply a soothing cream, such as tea tree oil, with a cotton ball to calm the area.

> **TIP:** *Numb the brow area beforehand with an ice cube or a dab of LMX or Anbesol cream.*

∾ Wax, Pluck, or Thread?

First of all, what the *hell* is threading, and why are people doing it? What does it *mean*? Is it some medieval torture-type thing? Sort of. It's an increasingly popular ancient Middle Eastern and Indian way of removing hair from your eyebrows, beloved primarily because it's so much quicker than tweezing (it takes roughly the same time as waxing: about ten or fifteen minutes total). An aesthetician will use a doubled-up piece of cotton thread to slide out the hairs from the roots, not touching the skin, which means less irritation (and potential wrinkles around the eye later on) for you. Whatever method you opt for, whether a novice or an old pro, the easiest option is to get your brows done professionally every couple of months, and then perform the tweezing upkeep yourself. Not only will it be less work, but a professional will be able to best assess what the correct brow shape for your face is.

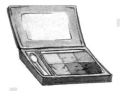

*Direct from Jolie in NYC:
How Long Will My Products Last?*

Q: *When should you throw out old products? I've heard you need to replace eyeliner and mascara every three months. But what about lipstick that's three years old? Or foundation that's two years old, and so on? I'm a product junkie myself, but my little bathroom is getting a bit overwhelmed with my collection.*

A: I find it nearly impossible to throw away old products, even when they're getting old, crusty, and crumbly. (Well, okay, it's *slightly* easier then, but still.) Unfortunately, being too attached to expired products can lead to breakouts and infections—not to mention the fact that your makeup simply won't look as good as it should. In general, mascaras will last three months, foundation will last for about six months, lipstick will last for a year, and powders (such as blush and eyeshadow) will last between one or two years. Toss perfume within two years—sooner if it's been in the heat or the sun. A good rule of thumb: liquid formulas (mascara, foundation) breed bacteria quickly, so they should be the first to toss. It's hard, but worth it—be brutal!

∾ Why All Mascaras Are Not Created Equal

Foundation and concealer are probably the most important, lip gloss the easiest, but ask women for the one cosmetic that they absolutely, positively could not live without, and the answer is almost always mascara. (Mascara, interestingly, is the beauty product often cited as having the highest consumer loyalty, meaning that when a woman finds mascara she loves, she's a fan for life.) Nothing else makes you look as awake, feminine, and sexy in such a flash. However, the choices—Lengthening! Curling! Thickening! Comb! No comb!—can be daunting, and actually applying the damn stuff properly is nearly impossible. The secret is in the brush . . . and in the formula . . . and in the wetness . . . and in the time since you've opened it . . . okay, you get the point. Getting perfect lashes doesn't have to be rocket science, though. The trick is to identify the type of mascara you need, then learn how to apply it correctly. (Oh, is that all?)

Lengthening: Okay, so it's essentially a no-brainer what the various mascaras do. Lengthening mascaras, um, lengthen. (Imagine that.) These mascaras tend to have wands with denser bristles, so they help pull the formula all the way to the end of lashes. Good for everyday use, as well as on special occasions.

Curling: I tend to be skeptical of curling mascaras, which use polymers that shrink to help pull lashes up (and stay curled once there . . . allegedly). Some people swear by them, however—people with lashes that are obviously more accommodating than mine.

Volumizing: These mascaras contain a thicker formula of waxes and silicone polymers that coat lashes and make them appear bulkier.

Waterproof: In a class of their own, because the ingredients that make them waterproof change the way they appear on your lashes. So, if you're obsessed with Mascara X, and then see that it's also available in a waterproof version, don't automatically assume it will appear the same on your lashes, as it might not.

Defining: This is a standard mascara without any bells and whistles, that simply takes what you already have and makes them darker and more visible. Don't confuse that with being boring, however. Some of the best mascaras in the world fall into this category, such as Lancôme Definicils.

∾ Mascara Tricks

▶ Product too clumpy? Run the (closed) tube under hot water to thin it out.

▶ When you pull the mascara wand out of the tube, wrap a piece of tissue around the wand and gently squeeze a couple of times to remove excess product. This will help ensure that the product doesn't flake or clump.

▶ Use an eyelash curler before applying mascara, not after.

▶ If you don't like the curl that an eyelash curler gives you, start at the tip of your lashes and work your way down (rather than the other way, as is normally advised), "walking" the curler down your lashes and gently holding it for about two seconds before releasing.

▶ For extra definition, or if your lashes are very faint, apply mascara both on the bottom *and* the top of the lashes. (This should not be confused with applying mascara on the bottom lashes under the eye, as this often leads to smudges.)

▶ For extra thickness, hold the wand at the base of your lashes and move it back and forth in a horizontal motion, as close to the lash line as possible, before pulling it up through the lashes to the tip.

▶ Toss mascara after three months. Some mascaras will start to turn as early as two months; you'll be able to tell that it's time for a new one when it starts clumping and is harder to apply than usual.

▶ If you are a blonde or a redhead, try brown or navy mascara, instead of traditional black, for a less harsh, more flattering look.

▶ Take an old mascara wand and rinse it clear of any residue, then keep it on hand to comb through dry lashes after applying mascara—this will help get rid of clumps.

∾ The List: Greatest Mascaras of All Time

Lancôme Definicils: The best-selling mascara from the brand that many regard as the best *producer* of mascaras, it lengthens and defines for a spidery look. Best of all, it doesn't flake or smudge. Not for the faint of heart!

Kiss Me Mascara: Goes on to form little "tubes" around the individual lashes for length and thickness. The coolest part? The tubes stay put until you want to remove the mascara (even if you cry or rub your eyes), when they then slide right off. A massive cult hit, and excellent for sensitive eyes and those who have problems with smudges.

Dior DiorShow Mascara: A glamorous powerhouse with a chubby brush that lengthens, thickens, volumizes, and separates. The only downfall is that it's occasionally prone to clumping. The famous rose fragrance, however, is divine.

Max Factor Lash Perfection: Features a special brush with comb-like bristles, to keep lashes from clumping while adding definition and length. Won't smear or flake, either.

Maybelline Great Lash: I have to be honest, this is my least favorite mascara—ever. It does nothing for my lashes, because it goes on very thin and watery, and gives only the slightest hint of color. For these very same reasons, however, women all over the globe adore it. (Let it never be forgotten that mascara is, indeed, a deeply personal thing!)

L'Oreal Voluminous Mascara: Does exactly what it claims to, which is to say, make your lashes appear thick and plump. The only downside is that, as with most volumizing mascaras, it can occasionally clump. Regardless, it's still one of the better drugstore options out there.

∾ No, It's Not A Torture Device— Why An Eyelash Curler Should Be Your Best Friend

Sure, it's an extra step, and no, you don't *have* to use a curler with mascara, but let's put it this way—I never use mascara without first curling my lashes. Ever. Just a few seconds on each lash, and your mascara will pay big dividends. Some people are blessed with lashes that naturally curl up and out, as if at perpetual attention. To those people, I say, lucky you. For the rest of us, lashes need an extra boost, and nothing makes you look more wide awake. My two favorite curlers are made by Shu Uemura and Shiseido: neither will pinch eyelids and both curl with just a couple of gentle clamps. Shu Uemura's version is better for round eyes; Shiseido is better for almond-shaped. To use, simply hold the curler at the base of your lashes and gently hold down for about five seconds before releasing and sliding the curler up your lashes a few millimeters. Repeat, slowly "walking" the curler up your lashes and being careful not to apply too much pressure. (Unless a crimped look is what you're going for; I assume it's not.)

How To: Apply Undereye Concealer . . . without Looking like An Albino Raccoon

Step 1: Concealers come in many forms: sticks, pots, pencils, cremes, etc. Pick whichever you like, but always make sure it's a shade or two lighter than your skin and/or foundation. If your skin is ruddy or pale, choose a light beige with some slightly pink undertones. Olive skin tones should look to a slightly darker shade of beige with yellow undertones. A medium-dark beige can be used for darker skin, preferably with peach undertones.

Step 2: Apply moisturizing eye cream. Make sure to apply it at least one inch below your eye, as cream travels up. Wait a minute or two for it to dry.

Step 3: Next, apply a very light amount of concealer under your eyes. Remember, start small—you can always add more, if necessary. Use a small concealer brush or your fourth finger (which exerts the least amount of pressure) to gently apply. (Careful not to wipe or rub, only pat—skin here is delicate and a little coverup now isn't worth the wrinkles later!) Make sure you blend with a soft touch.

Step 4: Add a small dab of moisturizer for a more translucent finish, and check the mirror. Smile into it to make sure nothing extra has gone into the little creases around your eye. Blot any mistakes with a tissue, and finish the look by using a small dusting of untinted face powder.

∾ The List: Best Under-Eye Concealers

Laura Mercier Secret Concealer: Available in three different shades (#1, #2, #3), Laura Mercier's Secret Concealer brings a youthful, bright look to the dark circles under your eyes. Dab it on with fingers or use a brush—these intense pigments are soft in texture, so a small amount is good to last. The moisture rich formula is perfect for dry, sensitive skin.

YSL Touche Eclat Radiant Touch: 3 in 1! The Radiant Touch pen is a concealer, highlighter, and airbrush wand together in one slim package. Sold in three shades (a pale pink, a light gold, and a warmer bronze), this concealer uses an optical light diffusing technique to hide imperfections and make your skin glow. It can even be used to camouflage blemished skin, or as a base for lips and eyes.

Smashbox I Prime Under Eye Primer and Concealer: Available in a wide range of skin tones from light to dark; this multi-purpose product offers both a primer and a concealer in a cute little case. The primer is used to smooth the skin, filling in lines and imperfections, while the concealer masks your dark circles.

Bobbi Brown Creamy Concealer Kit: Bobbi offers a healthy concealer: one that includes Vitamins A and E to condition and minimize wrinkles/dry lines while moisturizing under your eyes all day. Packaged in a little jar, the Creamy Concealer Kit includes a concealer on top and a sheer finish dust on the bottom. Choose from a variety of shades (twelve to be exact), smooth on concealer, dust on sheer powder to finish, and you're good to go.

L'Oreal True Match Super-Blendable Concealer: A serious bargain, this inexpensive oil-free concealer not only works for under your eyes, but can conceal blemishes and other facial imperfections. Also includes Vitamin E and Pro-Vitamin B5 to nourish and revitalize your skin.

Chapter Four Product Price Guide

$: less than $10
$$: between $10 and $24
$$$: between $25 and $49
$$$$: between $50 and $100
$$$$$: more than $100

Stila Kajal eyeliner, $$, *stila.com*
LMX, $, drugstores
Anbesol, $, drugstores
Lancôme Definicils, $$, *lancôme-usa.com*
Kiss Me Mascara, $$, *blincinc.com*
Dior DiorShow Mascara, $$, *eluxury.com*
Max Factor Lash Perfection, $, drugstores
Maybelline Great Lash, $, drugstores
L'Oreal Voluminous, $, drugstores
Shu Uemura Eyelash Curler, $$, *shuuemura-usa.com*
Shiseido Eyelash Curler, $$, *shiseido.com*
Laura Mercier Secret Concealer, $$$, *lauramercier.com*
YSL Touche Eclat Radiant Touch, $$$, *nordstrom.com*
Smashbox I Prime Under Eye Primer and Concealer, $$,
  sephora.com
Bobbi Brown Creamy Concealer Kit, $$$,
  bobbibrowncosmetics.com
L'Oreal True Match Super-Blendable Concealer, $,
  drugstores

Five

Complexion

Who needs an MD?
Becoming your own dermatologist

What do you see when you look at your skin in the mirror? Do you think, "Oh my God, I am *so* gorgeous"? (Hey, there, Paris!) Or do your eyes immediately zoom in on whatever "flaws" you may have, real or imagined? (Or, um, is this just me?) If you're under a certain age—let's say twenty-eight—whatever issues you have are likely of the "Why won't these zits go *away*?" variety. Once your thirties creep up on you, however, you start doing that thing where you pull out a magnifying mirror and study your skin *really close*, trying to determine if that line was there last week, or if a new freckle has suddenly popped up near your eye from too much sun.

We live in a youth-obsessed society, no doubt about it. Half of the models you see in top fashion magazines, strutting their underfed selves in items of clothing that cost more than my yearly rent, aren't even old enough to vote, let alone drink. Botox is practically a requirement in Hollywood for any actress over the age of twenty-five. And that glossy spread with the gorgeous woman who looks *so* unbelievable for her age? It's completely airbrushed. *People don't want to see wrinkles, you know,* whisper the art directors as they gleefully Photoshop to their heart's content.

It's no surprise, then, that dermatologists are the new beauty-world rockstars, worshipped for their nearly magical abilities to make skin—any skin, no matter what the condition —look movie-star perfect. Whether it's a cortisol shot to make a blemish disappear instantly, microdermabrasion, or a glycolic peel to thoroughly exfoliate and smooth skin, lasers to erase redness and discoloration, or Botox and Restylane to plump and erase lines, it seems there's almost nothing they *can't* do. Unfortunately, however, the services provided can be addictive, and are rarely cheap. Have ten thou a year to shell out on injections or intense pulsed light lasers? Good for you! As for the rest of us stingy paupers, we need more realistic options—after all, who has the cash *or* time to run to the derm every single time your skin flares up . . . especially when you can take care of it yourself at home? I'm spilling the secrets of all the Docs Hollywood right here. Thank me in twenty years—when you look the same age.

∽ What Causes Aging

I'll give you a great big hint. It's yellow and it lives in the sky. Surprise! It's the sun! This is the point where you roll your eyes and say, "Yeah. Duh," sighing to yourself about how beauty girls always dole out the same tiresome advice. I'm not

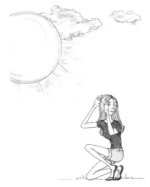

here to be your mother—believe me, I've made millions of beauty mistakes in my life, and if I told you I would never, ever again lie out in the sun at the beach, well, I'd probably be lying. But if you're one of the seventeen people in America who wears broad-spectrum SPF 30 or higher sunscreen, even when it's February, cloudy, freezing, and you're just running to the mailbox for fifteen seconds, then congratulations. You can feel smug. Everybody else? Stop smirking, because your skin isn't *nearly* as protected as you think it is.

Have I scared you yet? Or at least made you think, "Wait, what? What the hell is she babbling about?" Surely you want your skin to look the very best it can, no? You like it when your friends say, "Wow, you look so pretty!", right? It then stands to reason that you wouldn't *only* want those compliments now, and not, say, also twenty-five years from now. So, once again (sigh), here we go. I know you know it, you know you know it, but it can't be repeated enough.

No factor makes as big a difference in your aging prospects as the sun and environment. Your skin is made up of collagen and elastin (along with other stuff, of course, but this isn't a science lecture, so go check out a biology book if you're *really* interested), and when you're young, you have a lot of both. There are many, many factors involved in aging, of course. Skincare guru Dr. Dennis Gross, creator of one of my favorite skincare lines, MD Skincare, breaks it down very simply: "Aging is caused by the breakdown of collagen in the skin. As we age, skin's natural production of collagen slows and wrinkles begin to form." He continues: "Our skin has built-in natural defenses to protect it from damage, be it from bad sunburn, drinking too much alcohol, not sleeping enough, and a host of other things. Skin also has amazing regenerative abilities that help it repair any damage it may have incurred. But our skin also has natural enzymes that break it down. As we age, our skin's defensive and healing powers no longer outpace its natural degradation process. The net result is that our skin loses its ability to fend off and recover from internal and external stressors."

I'll never forget a beauty event I went to years ago where slides were shown of a case-study done with identical twins. One woman faithfully wore sunscreen her entire life, the other twin was a sun-worshipper and smoker. Side-by-side photos of the two of them at twenty were fairly unremarkable, but by the time the women were in their fifties, there could have been a fifteen-year age difference between them. The sun-loving twin's skin was noticeably browner, saggier, more wrinkled, and discolored. I think every single beauty editor there applied SPF 45 sunscreen the following morning.

Speaking of, what's the other great big beauty no-no? Come on, say it with me: don't smoke! Let's forget for a second the fact that smoking sends your risks of cancer through the roof. It also dries out your skin, causes wrinkles, and floods your system with free radicals (more on those later), breaking down your tissue.

But, you know, life happens—we've all been there. It's not practical to completely stay out of the sun, and if you get drunk with your friends and decide to sneak a cigarette, I'm not going to judge you. (Not to sound like a broken record, though, but—alas—your skin will.)

∾ Why the Term "Sunblock" Is Misleading

When you buy a sun product labeled "sunblock" or "SPF 60," you're not really getting what you pay for. Our current sunscreen label system is woefully uncomprehensive and uninformative. SPF 15, to pick a number, means that you're getting fifteen times the sun protection that you would if you didn't have any sunscreen on. Unfortunately, labels don't explain that the chemicals in sunscreen break down after a few hours, take between twenty minutes and half an hour to start working, and become virtually useless several hours after being applied, not to mention that you have to apply the recommended amount (one shotglass, or two ounces, for your entire face and body per application) and that most sunscreens only provide about half of the protection listed on the label. In fact, experts advise that you reapply sunscreen every *two hours*. The majority of us apply SPF 15 at about 8 A.M., and then forget about it, satisfied that we're doing a little something to keep ourselves looking young. By the time we head outside for lunch four hours later—when we'll actually be exposed to the sun for a significant amount of time, whether it's walking to a café, or driving to a lunch meeting—the sunscreen is basically ineffective. And take "water-resistant" and "waterproof": water-resistant simply means that the sunscreen's properties won't change for up to forty minutes of water contact; waterproof sunscreens only have to last eighty minutes. So, if you've been at the beach, swimming in the ocean for three hours, and you haven't yet reapplied, your skin is no longer adequately protected. As far as the term "sunblock," there is finally a movement to ban this incorrect term from labels—sunblock doesn't "block" the sun, period. It shields you from it, but it's not as if a layer of zinc oxide on your nose is the same as spending daylight hours chilling in a subterranean coffin. And research shows that anything above SPF 30 is essentially just extra moisturizer. (Although I *am* surprised that nobody's tried to market, say, an SPF 1000 yet.)

So what *should* you look for? There are two categories of sunscreen: chemical blockers and physical blockers. Chemical blockers absorb light and include PABA, Parsol 1789, avobenzone, and mexoryl. Physical blockers reflect light and include zinc oxide and titanium dioxide. Physical blockers are much less irritating to the skin, especially those with very sensitive complexions, and also generally provide better broad-spectrum coverage. As you likely know, there are different types of UV rays: notably cancer-causing UVB and wrinkle-causing UVA. If you're making the effort of putting on sunscreen, then please choose a brand labeled "broad-spectrum," meaning it screens out both UVA and UVB rays.

TIP: *It's generally accepted as fact that the current best sunscreens in the world are by La Roche Posay, including Anthelios XL and Anthelios L, a water-resistant, SPF 60 cream that includes highly effective UVA blockers Mexoryl SX and Parsol 1789 (Avobenzone), as well as powerhouse UVB blocker titanium dioxide.*

∾ Beauty Myth: Drink Eight Glasses of Water a Day to Improve Your Skin

Okay, I know you've been holding onto this one for years. Your mother drilled it into your head. You've read about it in magazines. Dewy-skinned celebs repeat it as their mantra and models stalk the subways clutching bottles of Evian and Poland Spring. But—please, take a deep breath here—there is absolutely no medical evidence to prove that drinking eight glasses of water a day does anything for you . . . other than send you to the bathroom every forty-five seconds. "Water levels are so closely regulated by the body that anything above what we need is urinated out," explains Dr. Gross. Of course, depriving yourself of water is unhealthy—nobody is disputing that fact—but overloading on it? Not necessary. Skin hydration is affected by many factors, including the level of the water content in your food and the amount of moisture in the environment. So, go ahead and have that glass of Pellegrino with your lunch. (Just don't feel obligated to have six of 'em.)

∾ Best Anti-Acne Products

Keeping those nasty, angry blemishes at bay can be a total nightmare. The only thing worse than pimples all over your face (or hell, even just *one* pimple on your face, especially when—surprise!—you have a seriously important event to attend that evening) is the flaky, embarrassing dryness that usually accompanies serious zit-busting remedies. Take heart, there *is* a way to make your complexion clear without looking like a shedding snake. Who knew?

Clean and Clear Persagel: With the strongest level of benzoyl peroxide that you can find over the counter (10%), this spot treatment will make pimples—even huge ones—vanish almost instantly.

Neutrogena Oil-Free Acne Wash: Something of a face wash miracle, since it doesn't dry out skin, even when used twice daily, yet still helps keep complexions in check. Only a few products are on my all-time, totally-in-love-with-'em list, and this is one of them.

MD Skincare Alpha-Beta Peel: One of the gold standard products adored by all beauty editors, these pads can be used daily to keep skin clear, exfoliated, and to help prevent fine lines.

Alpha Hydrox AHA Souffle 12% Glycolic AHA: Gets rid of breakouts, blackheads, and whiteheads, and helps keep skin smooth, plus promotes a glow. Bonus points because it helps get rid of wrinkles by increasing cell turnover.

Olay Total Effects Anti-Wrinkle/Anti-Blemish: The name says it all. Even better, it actually works.

Direct from Jolie in NYC: Could it be Rosacea?

Q: *I am in desperate need of something to reduce redness. Normally I just have really uneven skin but lately I am al-*

*ways red. I hate wearing full-on foundation but I look per-
manently sunburned! I called my dermatologist but my appointment is two months out. He is killing me but whatever.
Is there anything over the counter that works?*

A: I feel your pain; I, too, have a complexion that tends
to look tomato-red when left untreated. You might have
rosacea, a fairly common skin condition that causes skin to
flush when exposed to heat, sun, alcohol, stress, etc. (Basically, when exposed to life.) Definitely keep your appointment with your dermatologist, but in the meantime, there
are products at the drugstore that might help. Check out
the Eucerin Redness Relief line, Purpose Redness Reducing
Moisturizer with SPF 30, or (for something pricier but a favorite of many) B. Kamins Booster Blue Rosacea Treatment.
And not to be a total broken record, but you really should
consider Bare Escentuals i.d. bareMinerals foundation to
help cover your redness. It feels weightless on your skin but
covers redness like a dream (especially if you use the full
coverage kabuki brush) and also contains sunscreen. (A
note for those of you who have sensitive skin often irritated by sunscreens; physical sunscreens like zinc oxide and titanium dioxide—which is in Bare Escentuals—will normally
not irritate skin. It's chemical sunscreens, like Parsol 1789
or mexoryl, that cause more sensitive complexions to react
negatively.) I hope that helps until you can make it to your
derm! (See Chapter Six for more information on rosacea.)

∽ Your Genes Versus the Environment: Which Side Will Win?

Everybody's seen her: that girl who smokes like a chimney, drinks like a fish, subsists on greasy burgers and fries, lives in a big city, and sails through life, skin glowing like a newborn baby. This, my friends, is proof that somebody up there has a sick sense of humor.

Nothing will affect your skin like the environment you're in. People who live in Miami—or, for example, right under the ozone hole in Australia—are more likely to develop skin cancer than those who live in, say, Toronto. However, you can't discount the role that heredity plays in aging. Like 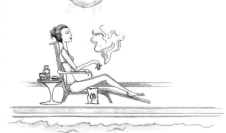 it or not, some people truly are blessed with great genes. Your natural face volume, the shape of your eyelids, the presence (or lack) of bags under your eyes—these are all determined by the cards you've been dealt. "It is impossible to separate the genes from the environment with respect to skin aging," says cosmetic dermatologist Dr. Kenneth Beer. "If you have bad genes and tend to wrinkle early but live in a place where you are not exposed to a lot of ultraviolet radiation, do not smoke, get a lot of rest, and use great products, you will look better than your years would otherwise dictate. If you have great genes but smoke, go to tanning beds, and live in the sun, you are going to wrinkle like a prune and there is nothing that some moisturizers are going to do to protect you."

As you get older, your face naturally begins to lose fat and volume in the cheeks, you get more wrinkles around your eyes, the nasolabial folds (the smile lines) and lines between your forehead begin to deepen, and bags often appear under your eyes and under your neck. However, the *extent* to which you're affected completely depends on genes. So, it really all comes back to that ancient standby: blame your parents. That, unfortunately, you can't change. What you can change is your environment. Soooo . . . load up on skin-saving ingredients like antioxidants, peptides, retinol, and hydroxy acids and wear broad-spectrum sunscreen.

∾ The Products and Ingredients You Need to Introduce in Each Decade

When you were young, you thought Corey Haim and Kirk Cameron were the cutest *ever*, but now your celebrity crushes are of the more rugged variety: Patrick Dempsey, George Clooney, Clive Owen, Brad Pitt (mmm, Brad Pitt). The point is, as you get older, things change: your tastes, your maturity level, and, of course, your skin. So, why on earth would you stick with the same products out of habit when there are doubtlessly other products better suited to your current needs? What worked at seventeen is probably not going to be the best for you at thirty. Sad, but true.

Your teens and twenties: Keeping your skin clear is of paramount importance, since your oil production is at its highest and you're likely to be suffering from acne. The two most important things you can do? Cleanse thoroughly and apply sunscreen. No matter how tired you may be, if good skin is your goal, please don't go to bed with makeup on. (Note: some girls—you know who you are—take pride in the fact that they never wash their faces, claiming, "It's weird, but my skin actually breaks out *less* when I don't wash it!" This may be the case. Aliens might also exist. I have no clue on either count. All I know is that, in the majority of cases, dirty faces equal clogged pores.) Look for ingredients with antioxidants like vitamins A, E, C, and olive-leaf extract, and apply in the morning underneath your sunscreen to improve its efficiency. It might seem tiresome now when your skin's all young and glowy, but—trust me—a few seconds' effort every morning will save you a world of trouble as you get older. Once you're in your mid-twenties, you can start using eye cream, but be sure to choose a gentle formulation that won't irritate the sensitive area surrounding the eyes.

Your thirties: Wrinkles are your main concern at this age. They're not everywhere, but you're starting to see more and more fine lines and evidence of sun damage. (I don't want to say I told you so about the sunscreen, so, let's just say . . . nothing.) Continue to use antioxidants like vitamin C, but start introducing peptides and retinol into your regimen as well. If you haven't yet done so, you might also consider a trip to the dermatologist for baby's first Botox (only in areas where you need it, such as the creases around the eyes and the frown line in the middle of your forehead, not all over—the Madame Tussaud's look is *so* not attractive) and skin treatments such as dermabrasion or light chemical peels.

Your forties: Collagen production is slowing; that can mean deeper creases and enlarged pores. As your skin becomes less elastic, pores expand because the collagen fibers in the walls around them are diminishing. To combat this loss, choose products with boosters such as retinol. Noninvasive lasers like Smoothbeam can also help stimulate collagen production and fight wrinkles without downtime.

Your fifties: Look for moisturizers that contain hyaluronic acid. It brings water from the atmosphere into your skin, making it appear plumper and firmer. You're prone to redness and irritation, so look for soothing products that include green-tea extract. It calms the skin, and studies show it can help prevent skin cancer. For deep lines, you have the option of using fillers like Restylane. Another option is a deeper laser procedure, though this requires recovery time and there's an increased risk of side effects such as skin lightening.

Direct from Jolie in NYC:
Day vs. Night Moisturizers

Q: *I can't wait to try some of the lotions and washes you recommended recently. My skin seems to be similar to yours: seriously sensitive, but I still manage to break out—not to mention dry out! I'm always confused as to whether I should be using different products at night. If my day lotion has SPF in it, I don't like to use it at night. Any recommendations? What should a nightly beauty routine consist of?*

A: The whole SPF/night cream thing is so confusing! Even though there's little, if any, difference between most moisturizers marketed for A.M. or for P.M., I think it just doesn't feel right putting on "night cream" during the day, or SPF-infused moisturizer at night. Regardless, unless you have extra-sensitive skin that gets irritated by sunscreen, it's actually fine to use your day cream at night and vice versa. (So next time you go on a trip and forget a night moisturizer, don't freak out!) Night moisturizers are often slightly heavier and day moisturizers usually have sunscreen, but other than that, they're pretty much indistinguishable. That being said, there are so many excellent night products out there, why not pick one that's going to do something good for your skin? Some of my favorites: ROC Age Diminishing Moisturizing Night Cream, Kinerase Cream, IS Clinical Active Serum, Philosophy Save Me, and Neutrogena Oil-Free Moisture for Sensitive Skin. These products won't inflame breakout-prone skin, and (except for the ROC and Neutrogena, which are just great, non-oily moisturizers) will even help reduce breakouts, so you won't have to deal with that annoying "Okay, this cream has zapped my zits, but now I'm molting" experience common to so many acne-fighting moisturizers. As far as the general routine, keep it simple: a gentle cleanser followed by moisturizer—and that's it. (Toners are generally a crock of BS, unless you simply enjoy the squeaky-clean feeling. Then, by all means, tone away!)

∽ Why Standard Skin-Type Classifications Aren't Helpful

Skin-type classifications are one of my biggest pet peeves. Maybe if I were a gal with cut and dry, one-size fits all skin, I'd feel differently and would rejoice at the thought of an entire line of products devoted precisely to me and my cookie-cutter skin. But I'm not, and I don't have that type of skin, and I'm willing to bet that you don't either. Case in point: let's say you're twenty-two years old. You've outgrown the oil-slick horrors of your teenage years, but you still get random, though frequent pimples, especially in the week before your period. However, when you go all commando on your blemishes, your skin freaks out and gets insanely dry and flaky—and the zits are still there. Sound familiar? Let's try another one. You're in your early thirties. You're still a fun gal—you listen to Justin Timberlake, watch crappy shows on E! and MTV, and even check out MySpace and YouTube occasionally. You feel young, and your skin probably does, too. You're starting to notice a few lines around your eyes and on your forehead, though, and if you have one too many glasses of red with dinner, your skin (not to mention your head) pays for it the next day. All the anti-aging products at the drugstore, however, are way too heavy and rich for you, and often lead to—are you kidding me? At this age??—pimples. Or still a third scenario. You have sensitive, ruddy skin . . . with wrinkles . . . and with the occasional zit. How to win? The fact is, everybody's skin is different, and whether it's due to environment, stress, or simply harder living, we all increasingly have to contend with wrinkles *and* breakouts, well before the age we should be getting lines, and well past the ages we should be getting zits. It takes a lot of experimentation and trial and error to find the products that will work for you, but they're out there. I prefer a mix-and-match approach to skincare, looking for products and ingredients to target certain concerns. Below, some of the best products for various problems.

∾ The List: Best Skincare Products for Real Concerns

BEST CLEANSERS

If your skin is always red and irritated OR your cheeks are always tight and flaky, try Cetaphil: Dermatologists swear by it for good reason; it's gentle enough for even the most inflamed, reactive skin, and won't further dry out those with severly parched or eczema-afflicted complexions. Apply to wet skin and wash off, or apply to dry skin and then tissue off residue. It won't give you that "squeaky-clean" feeling that many crave, but it won't strip or irritate skin, either.

If you're always getting zits, try Neutrogena Oil-Free Acne Wash: This classic orange-colored gel contains salicylic acid to break down surface oil and treat zits, as well as prevent new ones from forming. It really works, but also won't dry out skin.

If your skin permanently resembles an oil-slick, try Shu
Uemura High Performance Cleansing Oil Fresh:
Okay, it seems counterintuitive. Treat oil with . . . oil? This
cleanser is a superstar, however, and is beloved the world
over for its amazing ability to remove every last trace of
makeup and oil without stripping or drying out your complexion. (Well-moisturized skin won't need to produce excess oil; harsh cleansers often, paradoxically, cause sebum
glands to overreact.) I didn't believe the hype about this
product until I tried it; now, I'm obsessed.

BEST MOISTURIZERS

If your primary concern is getting rid of existing zits
and preventing new ones, try Clean and Clear Oil-
Free Dual Action Moisturizer: Feel free to go to the
department store and spend three times as much on a fancy
moisturizer, but this straightforward, salicylic acid night lotion is super cheap and works better than almost anything
else on the market.

If you can't leave the house without makeup because
of pigmentation and spots, try Kinerase Cream: This
moisture-boosting cream also dramatically improves the
texture and appearance of skin (we're talking visible results), getting rid of pigmentation spots, evening skin tone,
reducing the appearance of wrinkles, and brightening the
complexion. Use for three months, and you will absolutely
need less foundation.

If you have acne *and* are starting to notice wrinkles, try **Bliss Sleeping Peel Serum:** Something of a miracle in a bottle, this serum firms wrinkles and brightens skin with vitamin C and amino acids, and also helps keep it remarkably clear, preventing new blemishes and banishing the red spots that remind you of past ones.

If your skin has lines, dullness, and sagging, try **ROC Retinol Correxion Intensive Anti-Wrinkle Care:** Just a pea-sized amount used nightly will help plump up skin and diminish the appearance of wrinkles by increasing collagen production and cell turnover (which means that your skin cells are exfoliating themselves more quickly, leading to fresher skin). As a result, it helps with pigmentation and dullness, as well.

If all you can think after you wash your face is "I need moisture!", try **Crème de La Mer:** While I personally don't think this cream is the miracle potion it's touted to be, it *is* undeniably one of the best intensive moisturizers in the world. For dry, parched skin, nothing is better, and I defy you to tell me you don't feel luxurious putting it on. (And, hey, if it happens to get rid of a few wrinkles, too? Fabulous!)

BEST PROBLEM-SOLVERS

If a zit erupts right before a date, try **Clean and Clear Persagel followed by hydrocortisone cream:** The one-two punch of this 10% benzoyl peroxide treatment (the strongest you can get without a prescription) followed by the shrinking effect of a hydrocortisone cream such as Cortaid will have your skin clear in no time.

If you have the most insane dark circles under your eyes, try Hylexin eye cream: The same company that makes stretch-mark cream/anti-wrinkle cream Strivectin put out this powerhouse eye cream, which really does work to banish even the most stubborn undereye darkness and circles almost immediately.

If you still have redness from a zit that disappeared two months ago, try DDF Fade Gel 5: With a potent cocktail of known lightening-ingredients hydroquinone, kojic acid, and salicylic acid, you're guaranteed to rid yourself of pigmentation and dark spots. (FYI: in Europe, there are concerns over the safety of hydroquinone, which could be linked to cancer and is banned in some countries. I've used products with hydroquinone in the past and nothing's happened to me yet, but proceed with caution.)

If your skin looks duller and more lifeless than a corpse, try Clarins Beauty Flash Balm: This cult gel instantly brightens and revives tired skin, helping it appear instantly glowy and refreshed. It's a favorite of celebrities, beauty editors, and makeup artists alike, and works well on its own or under makeup. Especially great for big-night-out events.

If you're heading to your fifteen-year high school reunion and want to look eighteen again, try Freeze 24/7: Something of a facelift in a bottle, this cream temporarily tightens and lifts skin, mimicking Botox to relax lines and produce a tighter, firmer complexion. It only lasts for a few hours, so you must decide for yourself if the price is worth it (it costs around $115), but for a short-term fix when you absolutely must look your best, nothing beats it.

❧ Sticking It Out . . . Or Not

Sure, this might sound like "no, duh" advice, but listen to your skin. Just because a certain product is touted on commercials as a miracle in a bottle while simultaneously being praised to the heavens by your best friend, your favorite magazine, and that celebutante does not mean it's going to work for you. If you've been using a product for a couple of weeks and have realized that, no, it's *not* your imagination, and yes, it *is* making you splotchy and zit-prone, it's time to change. Give it away to a battered women's shelter or charity, participate in the product swap on Makeup Alley, or just return it—most drugstores and department stores will allow this with a receipt . . . assuming the bottle isn't completely empty, of course!

❧ Choosing an Eye Cream

One day you're chugging along, living your life, occasionally wearing sunglasses and sunscreen, and then all of a sudden—bam! Wrinkles. Dark circles. Pigmentation. Puffiness. What the hell is going on? Well, for starters, it's not surprising that the area around the eyes is one of the first places on your skin that shows its age, since this skin is extremely thin and delicate. All kinds of things will cause problems to pop up here, from genetics (thanks for the raccoon eyes, dad!) to the sun (yesterday nothing, today a huge, stubborn spot of sun damage) to happiness (it is a cosmic joke that the more you smile in the course of your life, the more you use the muscles that cause the area around your eyes to whisker and wrinkle—hey, at least it's cute).

TIP: *When you apply eye cream, pat it on with your fourth finger, as it's the weakest and will exert the least amount of pressure on the delicate, easily wrinkled eye area.*

Direct from Jolie in NYC:
Are Serums Really Necessary?

Q: *What's up with these serums? Everytime I go to buy a cream, the salesperson lavishes me with serum or concentrated oil samples. What's your opinion, are they that helpful? What's wrong with just using my moisturizer? The salesperson tries to extol the virtues of changing my skin, rather than just the surface. Is this a crock? These serums are expensive!*

A: The truth is, serums really aren't necessary. Serums don't contain different, mystical ingredients—they're simply more concentrated versions of moisturizer. While they're nice indulgences (since they often feel silky and luxurious), and certainly are capable of doing great things for your skin, they won't make you look twenty-five when you're forty; a top-quality moisturizer can give essentially the same results. (And, by the way, if a salesperson tells you that a beauty product will actually "change your skin, rather than just the surface," she's getting into dangerous waters, since these products are cosmeceuticals, not drugs, and are therefore not FDA-regulated. If they want to claim that they will actually, literally, change your skin, they have to get FDA regulation and approval—which costs a lot of money and takes a lot of time. It doesn't mean they can't "potentially" change your skin for the better, but they're not actually allowed to claim it.) Anyhow, there's nothing wrong with just using your moisturizer, provided it's full of the right ingredients: look for moisturizers with glycolic acid (AHAs) or retinol, both of which will help retexturize and renew your skin and can help reduce the look of wrinkles over time. And if you're simply dying to use a good-quality serum that doesn't cost a bundle, check out the Olay Regenerist line—many people swear by it!

∾ What the Hell Is a Peptide? . . . and Other Skin-Care Definitions

Because knowledge is power, here are the ingredients you need to become intimately familiar with, as well as a glossary of other good-to-know definitions.

Allantoin—a plant extract used in creams and skin preparations to heal and soothe.

Alpha-Hydroxy Acids—AHAs are derived from fruit and milk sugars and work mainly as exfoliants, improving skin texture and minimizing fine lines. Used in chemical peels. Includes glycolic acid. Generally more irritating than beta-hydroxy acid.

Antioxidant—any substance that reduces damage from oxygen, like that caused by free radicals (see below). Foods rich in antioxidants, such as blueberries and pomegranates, can reduce cell damage. This may prevent or even reverse diseases caused by cell damage, and potentially slow the aging process. Used in anti-aging products. Notable antioxidants include vitamins A, C, E, co-enzyme Q-10, olive leaf extract, and lycopene.

Astringent—commonly known as toner; lowers the pH of the face after cleansing and helps normalize oily skin.

Benzoyl Peroxide—a popular acne buster that increases cell turnover. Causes dryness in some people, one of the most effective forms of acne treatment.

Beta-Hydroxy Acid—salicylic acid is the only beta-hydroxy acid. It also exfoliates skin, improving texture and diminishing pigmentation. Used in many anti-acne products. Makes skin twice as sensitive to the sun, so must be used with sunscreen.

Botanical—products made from plants.

Ceramides—lipid molecules that protect against moisture loss.

Chamomile—an anti-inflammatory ingredient (and a super delicious tea).

Emollient—soothes and softens skin.

Emulsifier—a substance added to a product to thicken it.

Free Radicals—one of the primary causes of aging, free radicals are unstable oxygen molecules that weaken cells, causing damage and leading to wrinkles. Antioxidants will help counteract their damage.

Glycolic Acid—once applied, glycolic acid reacts with the upper layer of the epidermis, weakening the binding properties of the lipids that hold the dead skin cells together. This lets the outer skin "dissolve," revealing the underlying, healthier, smoother, brighter-looking skin. Under the umbrella of alpha-hydroxy acids.

Glycolic peel—a peel using glycolic acid that thoroughly removes a thin layer of skin, resulting in a more youthful, even complexion.

Hyperpigmentation—the darkening of the skin from increased melanin production, caused by ultraviolet light from the sun or inflammation following acne.

Keratin—gives nails and hair their resiliency.

Melanin—the dark pigment in hair and skin. An increase in melanin, resulting from the sun or acne inflammation, can result in hyperpigmentation.

Non-comedogenic—products that won't plug or clog the

pores, so don't cause skin irritation or pimples.

Panthenol—also known as vitamin B5; used as a moisturizer.

Petrolatum—also known as petroleum jelly. Lubricates, moisturizes, softens, and soothes skin.

Peptides—peptides are simple proteins made up of a combination of amino acids acting as hormones or neurotransmitters. Used in cosmetics to cause certain responses in skin, such as increased collagen production.

pH—pH is an abbreviation for potential of hydrogen. In cosmetics, it measures the level of acidity.

Retinoids—vitamin A and all its derivatives.

Retinol—retinol is a type of retinoid that is especially productive at reducing wrinkles and diminishing acne. It exfoliates skin, stimulates cell turnover, increases collagen production, and minimizes pores.

Salicylic acid—the only beta-hydroxy acid, salicylic acid dissolves layers of the skin and is used for eczema and acne, psoriasis, callouses, corns, keratosis pilaris, warts, and dandruff. It treats skin by sloughing off cells, preventing pores from clogging up.

SPF—stands for sun protection factor. Sunscreen products have an SPF; the higher the SPF, the more protection you get from sunburn.

Tea tree oil—a natural preservative used in soap, shampoo, and skin care products to clean and disinfect.

Titanium Dioxide—a physical sunscreen blocker that reflects light; very effective in protection against UV rays.

Toner—removes traces of dirt left after cleansing and returns skin to its natural pH.

Vitamin A—an antioxidant that exfoliates skin, stimulates cell turnover, and increases collagen production.

Vitamin C—an antioxidant that increases collagen production and regulates oil glands.

Vitamin E—an antioxidant that increases cell production.

Zinc oxide—a physical sunscreen blocker that reflects light; originally used as a whitening face powder. Can also soothe and heal skin.

⤳ Shh . . . We Won't Tell

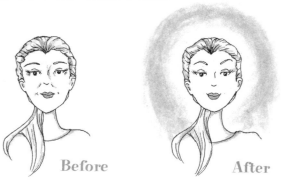

Before   After

Eventually, there will come a time when you can't improve your skin at home by yourself. That, my friends, is when you turn to the dermatologist for one of the increasingly popular cosmetic fillers and injections. Whatever your feelings on the increased plasticization of our society (hel-*lo Extreme Make-over*), the effect these procedures have on the skin is undeniable and immediate. Tiptoe into the waters carefully, however, because it's a slippery slope from "slight improvement" to "looks like she belongs in a wax museum."

Botox—the trade name for botulinum toxin A, Botox works by paralyzing the muscles in the face to reduce movement.

A few carefully placed injections treat a variety of problems, from frown lines in between the eyes, to those little whisker-wrinkles extending from the outer corners of the eyes to the temples, to the worry lines that pop up on the forehead. Contrary to what you might believe, Botox done properly and with restraint will *not* make you look frozen, only smoother. Botox also works well for younger patients who want to prevent wrinkles from increasing in intensity—the old "an ounce of prevention" theory.

Chemical Peel—a chemical solution improves and smoothes the texture of the facial skin by removing its damaged outer layers. Helpful for people with facial blemishes, wrinkles, and uneven skin pigmentation. Phenol, trichloroacetic acid (TCA), and alpha-hydroxy acids (AHAs) are used for this purpose.

Collagen—the most abundant protein in mammals and the main protein of connective tissue, collagen is commonly used in cosmetic and burns surgery. Injections can plump up areas of the body, particularly the lips.

Microdermabrasion—a skin-exfoliating technique that reduces fine lines and pigmentation. A sandblaster-like device sprays tiny crystals across the face, mixing gentle abrasion with suction to remove the dead, outer layer of skin.

Restylane—a dermal filler that restores volume and fullness to the skin to correct facial wrinkles and folds, such as nasolabial folds.

Sculptra—originally approved by the FDA to treat facial wasting and loss of volume in HIV patients, Sculptra is commonly used to plump up the skin to reduce the signs of fat loss.

✑ So, What About All Those Lasers?

Take a trip to your dermatologist's office, and you'll notice an increasing array of big, bulky machines with strange names that look vaguely like torture devices. These lasers are, no joke, the best thing to come along in years in terms of aging treatment and prevention. There's a laser for pretty much everything now, from wrinkles and fine lines to redness, rosacea, and broken capillaries, to hyperpigmentation and blemishes. There are even so-called "face lift" lasers, which dramatically tighten and tone sagging skin. And, of course, we finally have lasers to treat that teenage scourge: acne. Take a look at some of the most popular lasers to figure out which one is right for you.

> *Even beauties can be unattractive. If you catch a beauty in the wrong light at the right time, forget it. I believe in low lights and trick mirrors. I believe in plastic surgery.*
>
> *Andy Warhol*

IPL: Standing for intense pulsed light (also sometimes referred to as a FotoFacial), IPL is something of a miracle laser that treats seemingly everything: skin discoloration, acne scarring, broken capillaries, rosacea, fine lines, and unwanted hair (for more on this, see Chapter Ten). Depending on what you're trying to achieve, the wavelength of the light is altered, and melanin, hair follicles, or hemoglobin in blood vessels are targeted, allowing your body to go into repair mode to fix the injured tissue. Excellent for all ages. If your skin issues center around redness, choose the V Beam laser instead (see below); if you have a combination of redness and brown spots, the IPL is your best bet.

Cost: Around $300–$500 per treatment session.

Number of Treatments: At least three; six treatments for optimum results.

See results in: Three months; dramatic results in six months.

Pain factor: Mild to moderate. The quick laser pricks feel like rubber bands snapping against your skin for a fraction of a second. Hurts more around the nose and near eyes; often, one side of the face will be more sensitive than the other.

Downtime: None.

Lasts: Up to two years.

TITAN: This tightening laser for the face, neck, and stomach uses infrared light to make skin produce more collagen. It's also now used on previously difficult to treat areas, such as elbows, knees, and stretch marks. Best for women with noticeable but not excessive signs of aging, and not too much sun damage.

Cost: Between $1500–$2500.

Number of Treatments: One.

See results in: Three to six months.

Pain factor: Moderate. A brief, but hot, shooting sensation as the laser is quickly applied to your skin, then removed.

Downtime: None. You can head straight back to the office.

Lasts: It's a new procedure, so it's not yet known how long results will last.

SMOOTHBEAM: A firming laser, used for the face as well as the back, that also works wonders in helping to treat acne and acne scarring. It heats up the layers of collagen and sebaceous glands to kick up collagen levels (hence fewer wrinkles), diminish oil production, and smooth the skin from the inside out (never would have guessed from the name). Works well on women of all ages. Often used with V-Beam laser treatments to eliminate acne scar redness.

Cost: About $250 per session.

Number of Treatments: Six sessions.

See results in: Six sessions.

Pain factor: Moderate. Feels the same as IPL, but can be slightly more painful.

Downtime: None, although some people report bruising or redness on the face after treatments, or acne flareups before skin clears.

Lasts: Reduction of acne scars is permanent.

V BEAM: A gentle, pulsed-dye laser that's excellent at treating the redness and discoloration that goes along with hyperpigmentation, acne scarring, spider veins, and broken capillaries. Port wine stains and rosacea may also benefit. The laser shoots light onto the skin, which is absorbed by the blood vessels and then reabsorbed into the skin, eliminating redness and previously hard-to-treat issues like spider veins. If redness is your main concern, this is a better pick than IPL.

> **Cost:** It varies, since most doctors charge differently depending on how much needs to be treated.
>
> **Number of Treatments:** Three to six sessions.
>
> **See results in:** Two to four months.
>
> **Pain factor:** Mild to moderate. The same rubber band feeling as IPL (fun!).
>
> **Downtime:** None, although there is always the risk of slight redness.
>
> **Lasts:** Results vary.

THERMAGE: Heats the lower layers of skin and essentially "shocks" them, increasing collagen production (do we see a trend here with all these lasers?) and creating a visible, dramatic tightening effect in most people—which is why Thermage markets itself as the "nonsurgical facelift." It's effective on the jowly area under the chin, as well as the area around the eyes and on the forehead. Some people, however, report few results and feel it's not worth the pain or money. Also good for getting rid of cystic acne.

> **Cost:** Between $1000 and $5000, depending on how much of the face you treat.
>
> **Number of Treatments:** Typically, just one (some doctors may decide other sessions are necessary).
>
> **See results in:** One month for mild results, three to six months for more dramatic ones.
>
> **Pain factor:** Severe. Childbirth plus a gunshot wound to the eye plus smacking both of your funny bones at the same time . . . but only for a nanosec-

ond. Then, miraculously, the pain vanishes. Until the technician comes at you with the laser again.

Downtime: One day. Don't do this during your lunch break, as your doctor will probably give you a strong painkiller or relaxer to take before the treatment, and you'll feel loopy and sleepy afterward. Skin may have mild, easy-to-cover redness, like a sunburn, for a day or two, and slight swelling for a few days.

Lasts: You'll see results for about two years, if not longer.

BLUE LIGHT/LEVULAN: An acne treatment laser often used in conjunction with a photosensitizing drug called Levulan (the combined process is called photodynamic therapy), Blue Light is exactly what it sounds like—a blue light shined onto the skin that helps get rid of acne-causing bacteria, as well as dry up oil production and make the glands smaller. It will also help pores appear smaller.

Cost: About $150 per session.

Number of treatments: Two or three, with two or three weeks in between each session.

See results in: Two to six weeks.

Pain factor: Mild. You might feel a slight stinging, prickling, or burning.

Downtime: One or two days. Your skin will be extremely sensitive to the sun afterwards, so you must apply SPF 30 and remain inside the day following your treatment. Skin may turn crusty, but it's temporary and redness will fade in three or four days.

Lasts: For years; results tend to be extremely long-

lasting, although occasional maintenance is recommended as necessary.

FRAXEL: Fraxel treats wrinkles, sun damage, acne scars,
stretch marks, and fine lines by using thousands of tiny
laser spots to literally remodel the surface of your face,
chest, neck, body, or hands, leaving some skin untouched
to allow for faster healing. (Think of it as micro-pixelated
plastic surgery that airbrushes your skin.) Results can be
dramatic.

Cost: $1000–$1500 per treatment.

Number of Treatments: Two to five sessions, depending on your age and skin damage, ideally
spaced one or two weeks apart. Try booking the
last appointment of the day so you won't miss any
work.

See results in: Two to three months.

Pain factor: Moderate to severe.

Downtime: One day. You will likely not want to return to the office after your treatment, as your skin
will probably be red and slightly swollen. Over the
course of the week, your skin will flake and feel
sensitive. SPF 30 is a necessity for six months after treatment, and retinol and retinoids are to be
avoided.

Lasts: Years, however annual touchups are recommended.

∾ What to Do When You Head to the Derm

No matter what kind of laser procedure you might opt for, there are a few things you can do (and in some cases, must do!) to make everything go smoothly. Most importantly, if you've tanned or gotten sunburned in the past month, put away your beach towels, cancel your subscription to Palm Beach Tan, and go sit in a cave. Lasers pick up on the differences in skin pigmentation, and a treatment performed on your George Hamilton complexion will lead to permanent discoloration—not the look you're going for. Wash your face before you head to the derm's office, and take a mild painkiller at least thirty minutes beforehand, as well. Everybody experiences a different level of pain, so it's entirely possible that Thermage will be a piece of cake for you, or that IPL will be extremely unpleasant. Finally, wear sunscreen faithfully following the treatments, and be gentle to your skin for a week or so—no harsh scrubs, intensive acids, or spontaneous at-home microdermabrasion procedures. Be patient, too; it's normal to want results immediately—especially for the money you're paying—but recognize that your skin will slowly adjust and change over time, and that when you're finished with your sessions, you will absolutely see some sort of improvement. If your skin experiences any redness, try Lycogel foundation, which won't irritate post-op skin and draws oxygen into the complexion.

BEAUTY MYTH: Never Pop Your Own Blemishes

Technically, you're not supposed to pop your own zits—it's true that it does very easily lead to scarring, hyperpigmentation, bleeding, and unnecessary face-touching, mirror-staring, and "Why didn't I just leave it alone?" moaning. The truth, however, is that (shh) it is possible to pop your own blemishes, just like you've always suspected. Now, I'm not saying it's recommended, and when done improperly,

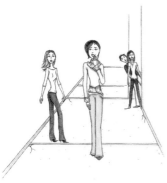

you could wreak some serious havoc on your complexion. But let's be real here. You want to do it. You're going to do it. So, at least do it right. First of all, never squeeze cysts—go for the white suckers just under the skin that are begging to be put out of their misery. Remove all makeup and wash your face and hands, to banish bacteria that might get into the open skin and cause an infection. (Optional steps: apply a warm washcloth to the skin for a few minutes, or sterilize a tiny needle with boiling water and rubbing alcohol and prick the surface of the skin ever so slightly. Personally, I never, ever go the needle route—I know people who have gotten infections this way. But I feel the need to mention that, if you are going to do it, then for the love God, sterilize it and be gentle.) Next take two cotton swabs or pieces of gauze and very (very!) gently press around the pimple until the white stuff surfaces and comes out, or when you see clear fluid. Don't press too hard—and never until you bleed!—because you could force the bacteria further into your skin, which will just cause a bigger, badder pimple down the road. (As for me, if I'm going somewhere soon after my minor bathroom-sink surgery, I dab on a tiny bit of hydrocortisone cream, to help the irritation and redness go down faster, then follow with a dab of medicated concealer.)

∽ Organic: To Be Or Not To Be?

When you think of the kind of woman who buys organic beauty products, chances are you think of some Birkenstock-wearing, Grateful Dead–listening, Berkeley-loving, progressive-causes-championing hippie chick. And, sure, there are doubtlessly plenty of those ladies (like my mother—love you, Mom!) buying organic shampoos and face washes and deodorants from fantastic lines like Jurlique, Care by Stella McCartney, Nature's Gate, Avalon Organics, Jason, and Cowshed. But there are also oodles (and I'm talking millions) of women just like you scooping them up, too. According to the consumer research group Organic Monitor, the growth of regular cosmetics has been flat over the last few years, whereas sales of organic cosmetics (and its natural cousins) have had double-digit growth. In fact, revenues will be breaking the billion-dollar barrier for the first time ever this year. Not too bad for a "niche" segment of the beauty industry, huh? But what does organic *mean*? What's the point of the products? Do they actually do anything? And, please—can they seriously be as good as "real" beauty products?

The answer is yes ... sort of. When a beauty product is called organic, it simply refers to the fact that the ingredients it contains are grown, manufactured, and processed in a way that is certified organic by the United States Department of Agriculture (USDA). This means no synthetic pesticides, hormones, or fertilizers, and no artificial colors or scents, among other qualifications. In order to bear the USDA seal, at least 95% of the ingredients in the product must have been produced organically. Anything less than that can't use the "USDA Organic" seal, however, many products will have, say 70% organic ingredients, and thus will still claim to be organic. So, interestingly, you could buy a product that claims to be organic, but which still has the same old chemicals and ingredients that you'd find in regular, nonorganic products. Kind of confusing, huh?

In any case, while some "organic" products are very similar —and thus produce similar results—to nonorganic products, most of the time, organic products will go bad easily and therefore must either be refrigerated or used before a certain date (two months is usually a safe limit). The fact that they're more natural, and perhaps less long-lasting, than other products doesn't make them better or worse, though—at least, not from the viewpoint of their efficacy. Your skin is porous and products placed on it can sometimes seep into your bloodstream (this is, for example, how nicotine patches work). So when you consider the mindblowing number of chemicals that you ingest during your lifetime, bringing down the number of potentially toxic things you put in your system is arguably better. As far as whether the products actually work, though . . . well, that's up to you to decide. Some people swear by organic products, others want their line-zapping and skin-plumping science and they want it *now*. I, personally, have been a fan of various organic products at one time or another, but have not yet felt the need to jettison *all* of my chemical-bearing products in favor of a natural, Whole Foods–beauty-aisle type life. My mother insists that my body will pay the price down the line . . . I suppose only time will tell!

CHAPTER FIVE PRODUCT PRICE GUIDE

$: less than $10
$$: between $10 and $24
$$$: between $25 and $49
$$$$: between $50 and $100
$$$$$: more than $100

Products

La Roche Posay Anthelios XL, $$$, *zitomer.com*
La Roche Posay Anthelios L, $$$, *zitomer.com*
Clean and Clear Persagel, $, drugstores
Neutrogena Oil-Free Acne Wash, $, drugstores
MD Skincare Alpha-Beta Peel, $$$$, *mdskincare.com*
Alpha Hydrox AHA Souffle 12% Glycolic AHA, $$, drugstores
Olay Total Effects Anti-Wrinkle/Anti-Blemish, $$, drugstores
Eucerin Redness Relief line, $$, drugstores
Purpose Redness Reducing Moisturizer with SPF 30, $,
    drugstores
B. Kamins Booster Blue Rosacea Treatment, $$$$, drugstores
Bare Escentuals i.d. bareMinerals, $$$, *sephora.com*
ROC Age Diminishing Moisturizing Night Cream, $$,
    drugstores
Kinerase, $$$$$, *sephora.com*
IS Clinical Active Serum, $$$$, *isclinical.com*
Philosophy Save Me, $$$$, *sephora.com*
Neutrogena Oil-Free Moisture for Sensitive Skin, $,
    drugstores

Cetaphil, $, drugstores

Neutrogena Oil-Free Acne Wash, $, drugstores

Shu Uemura High-Performance Cleansing Oil Fresh, $$$$,
shuuemura-usa.com

Clean and Clear Oil-Free Dual Action Moisturizer, $,
drugstores

Bliss Sleeping Peel Serum, $$$$, *blissworld.com*

ROC Retinol Correxion Intensive Anti-Wrinkle Care, $$,
drugstores

Crème de la Mer, $$$$$, *lamer.com*

Clean and Clear Persagel, $, drugstores

Hydrocortisone cream, $, drugstores

Hylexin, $$$$, *sephora.com*

DDF Fade Gel 4, $$$$, *sephora.com*

Clarins Beauty Flash Balm, $$$, *clarins.com*

Freeze 24/7, $$$$$, *freeze247.com*

Lycogel, $$$$, *lycogel.com* for locations

Jurlique, $$$, *jurlique.com*

Care by Stella McCartney, $$$, *sephora.com*

Nature's Gate, $, *natures-gate.com*

Avalon Organics, $$, *avalonorganics.com*

Jason, $, *jason-natural.com*

Cowshed, $$$, *cowshedproducts.com*

Experts

Dr. Dennis Gross, 105 East 37th Street, New York, NY:
212–725–4555

Dr. Kenneth Beer, 1500 North Dixie Highway, West Palm Beach,
FL: 561–655–9055

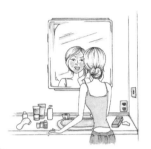

Six

Sensitive Skin

Your skin is not Mike Tyson; please don't beat it up

As a beauty expert, I'm supposed to know better.

Experimentation with products is all well and good, and variety is the spice of life, and if you don't mix it up, how will you ever learn what works for you? (And blah . . . blah . . . and blah.) But there's experimentation, and then there's common sense. In the mad, blind desire to determine the perfect skin regimen that will keep you looking twenty-five (No, twenty! Hell, why not fifteen?!) forever, sometimes even a beauty expert becomes a momentary fool.

This is my confession.

I'm in my bathroom, staring at my pores in my magnifying mirror, wishing desperately that I had a minuscule vacuum to suck out the nasty gunk. In a flash, the answer strikes me: Biore Pore Strips! Sucking out nasty gunk is what they were designed for, no? It is their *raison d'etre*. Lucky me, I happen to have an unused box of pore strips in one of my many trunk-sized suitcases full of makeup and skincare products.

Now, my skin is not exactly what you would call "tough"—sun, wind, and heat all turn me an extremely fetching shade of pink. I break out at the slightest provocation, turn purple after drinking wine, and once pussed for several hours straight after a particularly rough encounter with stubble. Sexy.

So, while the thought momentarily creeps through my mind, "But the last time you used the pore strips, they didn't take off anything but skin and you were left with a nose and chin that resembled a lobster for twelve hours," I disregard it. Obviously, lightning will not strike twice. This time, my pore strip quest for gunk shall be victorious.

Only, it's not. After I finish using the strips, I'm back in Lobsterville. And the gunk remains. And now I am angry.

Okay, okay. I can work with this. I need to get rid of this stuff on my nose and my chin. Exfoliation is key. If my skin were better exfoliated in the first place, the pore strips wouldn't have had any loose, excess flakes to grab onto, right? They would have immediately gone to the next layer and sucked clean the blackheads and whiteheads and sebum and grossness. And I wouldn't be faced with this problem now. It is *all* due to the lack of exfoliation. I need to remedy this problem immediately.

What's the solution? Well, duh. A glycolic peel.

Five minutes later, I am running around the bathroom screaming in agony, causing my roommates to poke their head around the door in concern, inquiring what the hell I've done to my face. Where there was once soft, pink skin is now a throbbing, oozing mound of flesh. I look like a pepperoni pizza. I feel like I have made out with a piece of sandpaper. I am less than pleased. Two Advil, an ice pack, and some hydrocortisone cream later, I am, at least, able to fall asleep.

The next day at work, I'm forced to explain to my boss, another beauty gal, what I did to my face. She stares at me in horror. "Biore Strips? And then a glycolic peel? What were you *thinking?*"

I don't blame the pore strips. (It's very big of me, I know.) Most people I know have had miraculous experiences with them, telling stories of pores vaporized and skin rejuvenated and complexions cleansed. The one-two punch of manual and chemical exfoliation, however, was obviously pushing it, particularly since I've been diagnosed with rosacea. In short, my skin is simply too sensitive for foolhardy "experiments." Lesson learned: sensitive skin needs special care.

But what is sensitive skin? Who has it? In the beauty industry, it's the buzzword on everybody's lips, new product lines devoted to sensitive skin are coming out seemingly daily, and more and more women are placing themselves in this category. Let's take a look.

❧ What Is Sensitive Skin?

Sensitive skin is more an idea that has become popular than an actual medical condition with defined parameters. In general, it refers to people who are allergic to certain ingredients in beauty products, as well as have skin conditions such as rosacea, eczema, and psoriasis. If your skin typically stings, itches, feels tight, or burns after applying products, it could be classified as sensitive. However, when it comes to having sensitive skin, the general populace suddenly starts channeling the old children's fairy tale "The Princess and The Pea": *everybody*'s skin is as delicate as a princess's bum. In the U.S., Europe, and Japan, roughly 50% of women label their own skin as sensitive. According to Eucerin, that number is even higher: between 50% and 60% of women.

While it might be trendy to jump on the sensitive skin bandwagon—after all, who wants to claim that their skin is "tough"?—there are a variety of legitimate conditions that necessitate special care for the complexion. So, if your skin flares up at the slightest provocation, or you've battled dryness or redness for as long as you can remember, it may not just be your imagination.

We'll take a look at specific, common skin conditions below, but first, a few good things to keep in mind regarding garden-variety sensitive skin.

▶ Choose products with as few ingredients as possible. Less ingredients mean less chance of your skin reacting negatively.

▶ Avoid products with botanical ingredients. Several botanicals, such as chamomile and rosemary, can irritate skin and aggravate eczema.

▶ Take care in extreme weather, such as snow, wind, or heat, all of which disrupt the skin's protective barrier and can irritate skin.

▶ Look for hypoallergenic, fragrance-free products.

▶ Wash your face with lukewarm water and never rub it dry.

▶ Stay away from harsh exfoliants like manual scrubs, or

irritating procedures like microdermabrasion and intensive glycolic peels.

▶ Always wear sunscreen with SPF 30. Look for ingredients like zinc oxide or titanium dioxide (physical blockers); avoid Parsol 1789, avobenzone, or mexoryl (chemical blockers), which could irritate your skin.

∾ Common Sensitive Skin Conditions, And How To Deal with Them

ROSACEA

You wake up in the morning and your skin looks fine, two minutes after washing your face, however, it's beet red. Or maybe your cheeks, nose, and chin flush after a glass of wine, or after time spent in a very hot or very cold room. Sound familiar? It's entirely possible that you have rosacea. According to estimates, rosacea affects a staggering 14 million Americans. (That's a *lot* of red faces.)

Rosacea—extreme facial redness often accompanied by stinging, roughness, and bumps or pimples—is as mainstream as skin conditions come, but the causes are still not known. It's believed to be hereditary, and the finger is usually pointed at blood vessels that dilate too easily. Rosacea often pops up in people over thirty, women going through menopause, and those with fair skin. Surprise, surprise: it's more common in women. (You're in good company, though; Princess Diana was a famous sufferer.)

Redness from rosacea tends to cluster in the center of the

face (the cheeks, nose and chin) or on the forehead, and typical characteristics include noticeable blood vessels, red bumps or pimples, and thick, rough, scaly skin. There are several different subtypes running the gamut from mild—a simple blush or sunburned look—to severe, which results in red, rough, and inflamed skin: one causes the stereotypical bulbous nose (here's looking at you, Bill Clinton!); another leads to watery, stinging eyes. It is estimated that between 50% and 60% of rosacea sufferers have some sort of eye problems, from mild issues like red or dry eyes, to light sensitivity, to major complications like inflamed eyes and even blindness. (Thankfully, this is rare.) Common things to avoid include detergents (wash pillowcases in dye-and-perfume-free cleansers, like hypoallergenic All Free Clear), perfume, and acids (such as glycolic and salicylic).

MANAGING YOUR ROSACEA

While there isn't a cure, there are many simple ways to manage and treat rosacea. The first step is figuring out what your triggers are and—imagine that!—avoiding them. Popular triggers include alcohol, spicy food, excess heat or cold (such as hot showers or saunas), wind, hot beverages, stress, and the sun. What does this mean? A life without margaritas, October baseball games, or pad thai? Not necessarily. By using the proper skin-care regimen, as well as considering the option of visiting your dermatologist for prescription creams known to lessen redness, you can enjoy most of the things you love . . . in moderation. (But if I see you on a hot, sunny day guzzling drinks in front of a wind machine, well, you're on your own.)

A little common sense goes a long way in rosacea management. Your skin is extremely sensitive, prone to dryness and overheating, and you're more likely to have eye problems. As a result, make sunscreen a religious part of your daily regimen (physical blockers, which reflect, rather than absorb, the sun's rays, are a much better choice than chemical blockers), avoid both drying soap and grainy exfoliators, and choose mild, hydrating cleansers. When eyes flare up, gently scrub with an eyelid cleanser or watered-down baby shampoo (yes, baby shampoo), then apply lukewarm compresses. And, of course, if your problem is serious or persists, see a doctor, who will prescribe steroid eye drops or oral antibiotics to treat eyes. Your dermatologist may prescribe Metrogel, as well as a sulfur cleanser, as treatment. Also, you may want to consider a laser treatment, such as V-Beam or IPL.

TIP: *Hot and flushed after exercising? Try sucking on an ice cube to cool down and lessen facial redness.*

HOW TO CLEANSE

Why do I need to learn how to cleanse? you might ask yourself. After all, you've been doing it since you were a toddler. (Or at least since you hit puberty and decided that hygiene was an important part of life.) I'm not pointing any fingers, I promise . . . but I'd be willing to bet that many of you are rubbers, scrubbers, and smushers, vigorously pushing cleanser all over your face in an effort to get *every . . . last . . . trace* of makeup, oil, and residue off. If your water is hot, and you were to complete this little complexion annihilation by, say, making out with a hand towel to dry off your face . . . well. Do I need to finish?

Your face is not your enemy. It loves you. It wants to look rosy and dewy and non-tomato-y for you. But you need to work with it. Slapping it around like an angry prison warden does nobody any good. Wash *gently* with lukewarm or cool water, and softly, delicately pat dry.

THE BEST PRODUCTS FOR ROSACEA

MetroGel: Your dermatologist will likely prescribe one of the MetroGel products typically used for rosacea management. MetroGel is for oily skin, MetroCream for dry skin, and MetroLotion for combination skin.

Cetaphil Cleanser: There's a reason this cleanser keeps popping up over and over; derms love it because it won't irritate sensitive skin. It may not be the "freshest" feeling product—because it's designed to be emollient, it leaves a thin film on the skin that many people don't like—but for easily-reactive skin, it's impossible to beat.

Purpose Redness Reducing Moisturizer SPF 30: The main appeal of this redness-calming product—other than the fact that it's simply another wonderful moisturizer from Purpose—is the fact that it's SPF 30; thank you R&D people.

Bare Escentuals i.d. bareMinerals: All mineral makeup is particularly helpful to women with rosacea, since it will cover redness without irritating skin. However, since I love Bare Escentuals, this is the line I use.

DHC Deep Cleansing Oil: Like one of my other favorite cleansing oils (by Shu Uemura; see Chapter Five), this olive oil-based cleanser removes all traces of makeup, but is very gentle and won't aggrevate rosacea breakouts.

Eucerin Redness Relief: This line includes a cleanser, daily SPF 15 lotion, green-pigmented tone-perfecting cream, and soothing night cream—the cleanser and tone-perfecting cream are especially popular.

ECZEMA

If your skin is severely dry or scaly, hot, itchy, and inflamed, you may have eczema. Also sometimes called atopic dermatitis (the most common form of eczema), eczema is a skin irritation, likely caused by the body's immune system overreacting to irritants, that often appears in infancy or childhood, then clears up before adulthood. (The National Institute of Health puts the number of people in the U.S. with eczema at 15 million.) Eczema ranges from mild, where skin is simply dry and itchy, to severe, leading to raw, broken, inflamed skin. It can be reduced with treatment, although skin will probably always be sensitive and need a little extra TLC.

As with most things in life, you probably have your parents to blame—eczema can be hereditary, although it's not contagious. Common eczema irritants include detergent, soap, dust, moisture, wool, and long baths. A recent study showed that mites in dust played a significant role in eczema; when the mites were reduced by controlling dust using Gore-Tex mattress covers, eczema was significantly limited. Other eczema triggers? Large cities (New York may be great for your social life, but it can certainly wreak havoc on your skin) and very dry climates.

MANAGING YOUR ECZEMA

First and foremost: do not scratch your skin! It's a vicious cycle, but the more you scratch or pick at scaly patches, the more irritated they'll become . . . and pretty soon you'll be reduced to slathering yourself in Crisco. (I kid you not. It's not the most glamorous treatment, but I know several people who have tried this. Even stranger—it actually works.)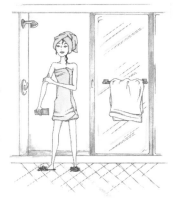

Your skin will desperately need moisture, so sleep with a humidifier and be sure to avoid hydration-sapping products like soap or detergents. While long baths, particularly those in hot water, can irritate the skin, short baths or showers in lukewarm water (with gentle, fragrance-free body wash, not soap!), followed within two or three minutes by emollient moisturizing creams, will help soothe mildly irritated skin. During more severe flare-ups, it may be necessary to see your dermatologist, who can prescribe steroid creams to reduce inflammation.

If traditional methods of managing eczema aren't working for you, consider seeing an alternative therapist, such as somebody who practices Chinese medicine. Sure, it sounds all hippie and hocus-pocus-y, but controlling eczema is about maintaining balance in the skin, and who better to help your body's largest organ find its inner chi? (In all seriousness, I know and have worked with many people who have, in desperation, turned to alternative therapists with astounding results. Give it a shot.)

> **TIP:** *Having trouble sleeping because your skin itches? Take an antihistamine; it'll reduce inflammation and help you nod off.*

BEST PRODUCTS FOR ECZEMA

Elidel: This steroid-free prescription cream, good for mild to moderate eczema, is sometimes prescribed by doctors.

Eucerin Aquaphor Healing Ointment: Thick and creamy, without being overly greasy, and hugely effective at healing and soothing dry, chapped skin.

Cetaphil Moisturizing Cream: A calming cream that sinks in quickly, but is too heavy for even slightly oily skin, so only use on the body if your skin is combination.

Cetaphil Cleanser: The one, the only, the classic. It's hydrating, emollient, and won't irritate skin.

Desert Essence Organic Jojoba Oil: A cult product available at health food stores, just one or two drops will moisturize the entire face. Bonus: you can use it in your hair for shine and softness, too.

Weleda Skin Food: An organic moisturizer that's extremely gentle and helps calm flakes.

Burt's Bees Buttermilk Lotion: With a baby-soft smell, this thick lotion is very emollient and is beloved by many.

Gold Bond Ultimate Healing Skin Therapy Lotion: Treats cracking skin by helping to fill in breaks.

Crisco: Works wonders in a pinch. I know plenty of people who have used this, and it really does soothe and moisturize dry skin.

PSORIASIS

Affecting over 9 million people, psoriasis is an immune disease affecting skin and joints that causes patches of thick, red skin with silvery scales, known as plaques. The cause is not entirely known, but for some reason, the body begins producing excess skin that flakes off more rapidly than during a normal skin cycle, often on the elbows, knees, scalp and lower back—although it can effect the entire body. Though psoriasis is not contagious, there is no cure and sufferers have a long history of being maligned. In the 1960s, a famous advertising campaign depicted "The heartbreak of psoriasis," while until the nineteenth century, psoriasis was frequently seen as a type of leprosy. Several factors contribute to psoriasis, such as stress, alcohol, smoking, obesity, strep throat, and climate or seasonal changes. Psoriasis is hereditary for about 30 percent of sufferers.

MANAGING YOUR PSORIASIS

The build-up of skin often goes hand-in-hand with excessive dryness, so the most effective psoriasis treatments will take a step-by-step approach to reduce inflammation while hydrating and soothing it. Traditional remedies include prescription ointments and creams, sometimes used in combination with over-the-counter products containing salicylic acid, or oral medications, while photodynamic light therapy is also very popular. Studies have shown that short, non-burning stints of exposure to UVB rays help treat psoriasis. I'm not advocating moving to Brazil and buying at-home tanning beds, but very small doses of exposure to natural sunlight a few times a week will likely be beneficial. (Too much sun, however, could trigger an outbreak, so tread with caution.) Bathe daily in lukewarm water with epsom or dead sea salts, oatmeal or apple cider vinegar to help soothe skin and remove scales. As with eczema, some people have found homeopathic medicine to be very helpful in balancing the body and controlling outbreaks.

BEST PRODUCTS FOR PSORIASIS

Epsom Salts: Add to a lukewarm bath and soak for fifteen minutes to help reduce itching.

Dead Sea Salts: Like epsom salts, dead sea salts are extremely effective to calm and soothe irritated skin. The high concentration of bromides in dead sea salts is thought to be a factor.

Neem Oil: Incredibly moisturizing, with ancient healing properties that many claim are a secret weapon for psoriasis (if you believe in that sort of thing . . .).

Coal Tar: Used for centuries, coal tar can be bought over-the counter and works well to reduce symptoms with no side effects, although it's still not understood exactly *why* it works.

Tazorac: A topical retinoid that your doctor can prescribe you, Tazorac was formulated for people with psoriasis and works by normalizing your skin's DNA activity.

Flaxseed or Fishseed Oil Capsules: Both contain omega–3 fatty acids, found in fish, which are good fats that help keep skin hydrated and healthy, and aren't naturally produced by the body.

Cortisone Cream: Over-the-counter cortisone creams will help reduce inflammation and temporarily soothe irritated skin.

TIP: *If you enjoy natural remedies, apply olive oil to your skin immediately after bathing to help moisturize.*

CHAPTER SIX PRODUCT PRICE GUIDE

$: less than $10
$$: between $10 and $24
$$$: between $25 and $49
$$$$: between $50 and $100
$$$$$: more than $100

Metrogel, $$$, *metrogel.com* for dermatologists
Purpose Redness Reducing Moisturizer SPF 30, $,
   drugstores
Bare Escentuals i.d. bareMinerals, $$$, *sephora.com*
DHC Deep Cleansing Oil, $$$, *dhccare.com*
Eucerin Redness Relief, $$, drugstores
Elidel: $$$, *elidel.com* for dermatologists
Eucerin Aquaphor Healing Ointment, $, drugstores
Cetaphil Moisturizing Cream, $, drugstores
Cetaphil cleanser, $, drugstores
Desert Essence Organic Jojoba Oil, $$, *desertessence.com*
Weleda Skin Food, $$, *usa.weleda.com*
Burt's Bees Buttermilk Lotion, $, *burtsbees.com*
Gold Bond Ultimate Healing Skin Therapy Lotion, $,
   drugstores
Crisco, $, grocery stores
Epsom Salts, $, drugstores

Dead Sea Salts, $, drugstores

Neem Oil, $, organic health food stores

Coal Tar, $, drugstores

Tazorac, $$$, *tazorac.com* for dermatologists

Flaxseed or Fishseed Oil Capsules, $$, health food stores

Cortisone Cream, $, drugstores

Seven

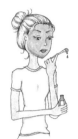

Face

Your skin is the palette and you are the artist—have fun with makeup

Think back to when you were about twelve or thirteen and a few girls in your grade began wearing makeup. Do you remember that one girl—let's call her Jenny—who sported a layer of orange foundation so heavy it literally looked like a mask? Poor Jenny was disregarding the cardinal rule of foundation: it must look natural. Otherwise, what's the point? Now, obviously, if you're wearing foundation, it's because you think you've got something to hide: redness, blemishes, unevenly pigmented skin, whatever. But twenty layers of face paint—particularly when it's the wrong color—completely defeats the purpose. And if you can see an actual line of demarcation along the jaw (here: orange; there: pale), that's just not right.

It's easy for me to point fingers now that I'm *so* much older and wiser, but it took me years of trial and error to settle upon a makeup look I'm comfortable with. When I was twelve, my family and I moved from Dallas to Atlanta. Despite my pleas and protestations and threats, my parents refused to let me wear makeup like all the other girls in my class, thereby subjecting me to life as a perennial outcast, doomed to roam the halls forever, pointed and laughed at by the other, prettier, more makeup-ed girls. (Or, at least, that's how it seemed in my young head.) After weeks of complaining and sighing, I finally wore them down, and they reluctantly agreed that I could wear makeup—*if* (and it was a big "if") I could bring home straight A's on my report card.

I have never studied harder in my life.

On that fateful day, the day I was becoming a woman (A woman! Finally!), my mother took me to the Clinique counter at our local Macy's for initiation into that secret club: the Clinique 3-Step Skincare System. To this day, I am unable to see that familiar yellow bottle of moisturizer, sliding tub of soap, or purple jar of watery lotion without remembering how happy and proud I felt. Not only was I getting to wear makeup; I was getting a *skincare regimen*, too. This was big-time.

After we got the skincare out of the way, we got down to the real business of foundation, the thing which my heart craved above all other. Not knowing in 1992 at the age of twelve what rosacea was, I only knew that I'd been cursed my entire life with a Rudolph nose and a ruddy chin, and I wanted them gone. Foundation was the way, the answer, the truth, the light. The saleslady blended shades into her wrist and my chin, buffing and blotting until she found the magical foundation color that was destined to make me look as beautiful as Christy Turlington or Jennie Garth or Mariah Carey. Once I had my precious foundation, I glopped it on, and never looked back.

Until, that is, I was twenty-two, a beauty assistant at *Lucky* magazine, and finally allowing myself to admit the awful truth: I hated my foundation. I couldn't find one that worked. *My foundation looked terrible on me.* The brand was irrelevant, and in any case, I think I switched brands every other month, in the hope that *this* time, I would find the miracle pill that would not only hide redness, but also not make my skin breakout, not feel like I was wearing dirt on my face, not be impossible to remove at night, and not look like I was wearing a mask.

Then one day, I stumbled onto it—my miracle foundation. It exists! No redness, no cakiness, no mask-like dirtiness, no makeup-induced breakouts; only clean, fresh, clear-looking skin. (My brand, in case you are wondering, is Bare Escentuals, my absolute, positive, cannot-leave-home-without-it love—see below.) I now refuse to change, occasionally testing out other waters only to snap right back home like a rubber band, faithfully declaring loyalty to my brand until the day I die.

The point is, it might seem like just *foundation*—I mean, please, whatever—but there is one out there that will make you look like you were sprinkled with fairy dust and blessed by the skin gods on the day of your birth. It's out there. I've seen the promised land, and it has flawless cheeks.

∾ Finding the Right Foundation for You

Step 1) Coverage

Start by figuring what level of coverage you need. Most magazines, particularly in the summer, advise dabbing on a hint of tinted moisturizer—and voila! Now, I don't know about you, but my skin does not look like a supermodel's. Thankfully, I've never experienced debilitating acne, but I'm definitely prone to a breakout or three and have a mild case of rosacea. With a permanently pink nose and lingering spots on my chin as a reminder of zits past, the thought of "tinted moisturizer—and voila!" is laughable. Coverage is a necessity. Luckily, modern foundations run the gamut from barely-there to kabuki-mask-heavy in a variety of shades designed to meld with any skintone. Deciding how much coverage you need will influence the kind of foundation you pick. Blessed with perfect skin? (Darn you.) Pass directly to Go, collect $200, and buy some tinted moisturizer in the process. Is your complexion good most of the time, with only a few minor, occasional imperfections? The foundation world is your oyster: you could go with tinted moisturizer on normal days, with liquid or powder foundation applied only where and when needed. Slightly fussy skin? Forget the tinted moisturizer—you'll need either a liquid, powder, or cream foundation (we'll figure it out below, based upon your skin type). Finally, if your skin is something of a problem—i.e., you have severe acne, or perhaps a skin condition like vitiligo—you'll want a specialty, heavy-coverage foundation such as DermaBlend.

Step 2) Formula

Now that you've determined what level of coverage you need, it's time to decide upon a formula: liquid, cream, or powder?

Here, an easy cheat sheet:

If your skin is DRY:
Use a moisturizing liquid or cream foundation with special hydrators for dry skin.

If your skin is NORMAL/DRY:
Use a liquid or powder foundation.

If your skin is NORMAL/OILY:
Use an oil-free liquid foundation or a powder foundation.

If your skin is SENSITIVE OR ACNE-PRONE:
Use a mineral-based, talc-free powder foundation specifically designed not to irritate skin or clog pores.

Liquid: The high-school cheerleader of foundations, liquid formulations tend to be the most popular, with the most ingredients and options—Oil-free! Anti-acne! All-day wear! Liquid foundations are the most likely to disappear right into your skin (figuratively, of course, 'cause literally would just be freaky).

Cream: Cream foundations are especially effective for gals who need serious, heavy-duty coverage. The upside is that your skin will look flawless, like you've never even heard of the word blemish. The downside is that the base will likely *not* feel natural, as it's kind of difficult to feel natural when you have hard-core paint slathered all over you. You win some, you lose some.

Powder: While not all forms of powder foundation are also made of minerals, this is the biggest growing segment of foundations right now. Whether mineral or not, powder foundations tend to be better for slightly oilier skins that may not like the feel of a heavier liquid or cream. The downside, however, is that powder foundations can magnify pores or fine lines, and can make some skin types (usually drier complexions) look too matte. Avoid powders with talc if your skin is sensitive or acne-prone.

Step 3) How to Apply

Carol Shaw, celebrity makeup artist and creator of LORAC makeup, advises using a sponge (or even fingers) to get the most natural, non-mask-like coverage. Across the board, makeup artists agree that foundation is only necessary where you actually need it. That is to say, if your t-zone always looks slightly discolored, but you have perfectly even cheeks, don't feel it's necessary to glop makeup everywhere—just be sure to apply with a light touch and then blend well. If you want a flawless finish, however—say you're going to be photographed, are heading to a special event, or simply feel that you're having a really, really bad skin day—Carol Shaw advises applying foundation with a makeup brush, starting in the middle of your face and working out.

∾ Application Method

Fingers: For under eyes apply concealer with finger tips and lightly (very lightly) dust a translucent powder on top to lock down.

Brush: Delivers the most flawless finish while also using up the least amount of foundation. Dip the brush into your foundation—a little goes a long way!—and smooth into skin, beginning in the center of your face.

Sponge: Put the sponge on top of the foundation bottle and turn it upside to shake a small amount out, then pat it over your skin, making sure to get in between the crevices between your nose and the area around your eyes.

> **TIP:** *Jerrod Blandino, creator of Too Faced Cosmetics, warns against trying to use foundation that's darker than your skin tone to achieve a tan. "This looks very 80s—you might be cast in the next* **Dynasty** *reunion show," he quips. A better option? Bronzer or self-tanner.*

∽ Why I'm So Obsessed with Bare Escentuals

I'll admit it, I have an obsessive personality. I don't just like tomatoes. I *love* them and eat them every single day. I didn't think Matt Davis was just *kinda* cute in eighth grade. I knew—knew!—he was the awesomest, coolest, most fabulous boy in the school—no, the universe!—*ever* and wanted to know anything and everything about him and be with him for all eternity. I don't enjoy Pearl Jam casually. They are my favorite band of all time and I am besotted by them and they will be the soundtrack of my life until the day I die. *Arrested Development?* Funniest show in the history of television, comedy, the world. Period. End of discussion.

Point is, I'm kind of a weirdo.

There is one thing I'm obsessed with, however, that I can

take comfort in, as it's neither random, nor quirky, nor nonsensical. That would be, of course, Bare Escentuals i.d. bareMinerals, my foundation of choice. For somebody like me, for whom "no foundation" is simply not an option, I need coverage to hide my red nose, ruddy cheeks, pigmentation scars, and uneven skin tone. The big problem with this, though, is that I absolutely *hate* foundation. I mean, it feels like you're slapping dirt all over your face, and then all day long it's fading and sweating and rubbing off on things it shouldn't be rubbing off on and just generally making you feel like you're wearing a mask. And if your skin breaks out easily, it's the absolute worst. It's a catch 22 because the more zits and redness you have, the more you want to cover them up. More coverage, however, equals more zits! How on earth can you win? There are, of course, foundations with anti-acne medication like salicylic acid, but I still can't shake that dirty, paint-on-my-face feeling. So, when I discovered Bare Escentuals, I felt like it had been created *just for me.* Not only does it feel like absolutely nothing's on your skin, which is a miracle in itself, it also wonderfully, perfectly covers redness and zits and all that gross stuff. It is, in short, my favorite beauty product ever and something I simply can't live without. Dreams do come true.

TIP: *Discard foundation every three months to avoid bacterial growth that can clog pores and cause breakouts.*

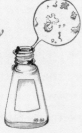

∾ Concealer

While foundation might be the main show, concealer is the cult act on the second stage with the hard-rockin' mosh pit. Like a brilliant mascara, concealer is one of those products that inspires feverish devotion or passionate anger—you'll either love a particular formula and what it does for your skin, or hate it. Not all concealers are created equal, and depending on what you're looking to cover, you'll need to seek out very different things. We've already covered undereye concealers (see Chapter Four), which tend to be slightly more emollient than concealers for pimples and scars. If you *are* trying to cover a pimple or scar, look for a heavier, drier concealer to better hide the problem without letting skin shine through, and always apply before foundation.

> *I'm tired of all this nonsense about beauty being only skin-deep. That's deep enough. What do you want, an adorable pancreas?*
>
> *Jean Kerr*

∾ The List: Best Concealers

Laura Mercier Secret Camouflage: With two different tones (one slightly more yellow-based, one more pink), it's easy to mix and match to ensure you get the perfect shade of coverage and to hide redness. The formula is drier than

Laura Mercier Secret Concealer, giving it great sticking power.

Yves Saint Laurent Touche Éclat Radiant Touch: We mentioned this bestselling product earlier as great for eyes, but these same highlighting properties also make it excellent for concealing small pimples and redness.

L'Oreal Paris True Match Super-Blendable Concealer: I don't understand the technology—something about changing to perfectly mimic your skin's shade and texture —but I also don't really care, simply because it works (yep, for both undereyes and pimples).

Dermablend Smooth Concealer: Super-heavy and opaque, this is the go-to concealer for when you need serious (and I mean *serious*) coverage.

∽ How To: Look Gorgeous (And Shine-Free!) in Photographs

Have you ever noticed that no matter how fabulous your reflection in the mirror may be, as soon as somebody whips a camera out, it looks like you've dipped your face in a tub of Vaseline? The camera flash has a way of illuminating shine that's barely visible to the naked eye. In fact, on photo shoots, next to the camera stands a minion whose *only* job is to rush in every two minutes and reapply powder to the star's mug— that's how serious this shine-free business is, people. For us plebians, a special

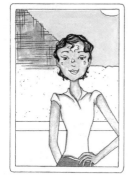

shine-zapper trailing after you isn't necessary, as long as you take the right steps before a big, photo-friendly event.

Step 1: Prep skin by washing face, gently patting dry (so as not to aggravate skin), and applying oil-free moisturizer.

Step 2: Apply a makeup primer to your T-zone, focusing on the forehead, chin, and nose. Primers (popular versions include Smashbox, Laura Mercier, Trish McEvoy, and OC8) will sop up oil and help prevent your skin looking greasy.

Step 3: Use a makeup sponge or brush (your fingers will only add oil to your face) to apply oil-free (are we seeing a trend here?) foundation and concealer. (Celebrity makeup artist Elke Von Freudenberg advises against using mineral makeup, which can be too shiny and reflective under the camera flash.)

Step 4: Finish skin with a light dusting of translucent loose or compact powder. If you're going out for the evening and can bring it with you, slip the powder into your purse and—after dabbing skin with oil-blotting papers—(very lightly!) reapply every hour or two. MAC Blot is an excellent oil-blotting compact powder. (Note: avoid putting powder on your cheeks, which can look cakey. Stick to the T-zone for best results.)

∾ Self-Tanner

BUT IT MAKES MY FACE LOOK ORANGE! WHY THE RIGHT SELF-TANNER WILL DO WONDERS FOR YOUR LOOKS

We'll cover self-tanners in depth in Chapter Nine, but it bears repeating, because whoever invented this stuff is a serious genius. While it may not be an actual, verifiable *fact* that self-tanner makes your face look prettier, healthier, and thinner, it's accepted as truth in the beauty world. Think about it—do you remember the last time you took a vacation to Florida or the Bahamas and came back with a slightly pink nose, and a golden bronze complexion? Now, do you remember all the compliments that this particular look brought you? Exactly. For whatever reason, our society has decided that being tan = being prettier, with few exceptions. (There are *always* exceptions. Many people can—and do—go way, way overboard on the color. For the love of God, let Donatella Versace be a warning to you!) It does kind of make sense; the darker your complexion, the less light bouncing off your face, and so the smaller it appears . . . maybe? Anybody? Well, regardless, try it for yourself. Dip into one of the new moisturizers with a hint of self-tanner for a week (these typically contain a mixture of old-school DHA and new-school erythrylose, as opposed to for-experts-only DHA-exclusive tanners, which can produce George Hamilton–type disasters in the hands of beginners), and I defy you to tell me that you don't notice a difference . . . a spring in your step . . . a sudden desire to, like, you know, totally go to the beach and wreck your hair with Sun-In.

∾ Choosing a Blush

It amazes me how many women sail through life either wearing the wrong shade of blush, or not wearing it at all ("No, no, thank you, my cheeks and nose are too red for *that!*"). In actuality, there is a blush for everybody, and all women can benefit from finding the best blush for their complexion. Blush warms up your face, brings out your cheekbones, and makes you look younger . . . not to mention can impart a certain naughty glow that brings other things to mind. Hey, I'm just saying . . .

Powder: Old school blush is still, objectively speaking, probably the most popular, and you can find a shade to suit absolutely any complexion. The better the formula is, the longer it'll stay on your skin without fading, and this is the easiest method to control the amount of blush applied. In general, powder is best for those with oily skin.

Cream: Tends to be more popular with younger women who want a dewier, more natural look, but the disadvantage of cream blush is that it can fade, crease, and smudge easily, especially in heat. When applied sparingly and properly, however, it can create a gorgeous, lit-from-within Botticelli goddess look that's unparalleled.

Liquid: Lasts for ages, and won't smudge at all. It can be hard for beginners to master, because it sets immediately and it takes a while to learn how much to apply (too much makes your face look like a red inkblot; not enough and you simply have weird dots on both sides of your face).

Gel: Gel blush, while not as popular as the other types, is long lasting and smooth to apply. Use your fingers and optionally seal with powder on top.

∾ How To: Apply Blush

Forget that stripey old 80s technique, which, rather than "creating cheekbones," will only serve to make you look like an extra in a Robert Palmer video. Instead, focus on the apples of your cheeks, lightly brushing back and down toward your ear to shadow your face, which will, in turn, emphasize your cheekbones. If you're using cream or liquid, simply dot a small amount of the blush on the apples of your cheeks and blend well.

> **TIP:** *I like to apply my blush last—after mascara, lipstick, everything. This ensures you don't put on too much and simply lets the blush act as a finishing tool to brighten your face and give a subtle, sexy flush.*

∾ The List: Best Blushes

Benefit Benetint: Famously created for strippers who wanted something that would effectively tint their nipples pink without rubbing or sweating off, this cultish stain works on both cheeks and lips to give you the prettiest flush this side of . . . well, really naughty things, such as strippers with blush on their nipples.

NARS Orgasm: Is there a reason this blush is name-checked, like, seventy-five times in this book? Oh, yeah. That's because it's insanely flattering and looks good on absolutely anybody. Right.

Benefit Dandelion: Now, it's not that Benefit and NARS actually hold the patent on phenomenal blushes . . . but seriously, what kind of magic are their research and development departments up to? This is a peachy, subtle blush that also works on just about everybody and warms up your complexion as if by magic. Better for daytime and the office, or when you've got a lot of other makeup going on at night and want something pretty and flattering that also won't compete with the rest of your look (read: give you Hooker Face).

Smashbox O-Glow: A why-hasn't-anybody-created-this-sooner? gel that reacts differently on everybody to turn your cheeks the exact shade they are when you flush normally. Revolutionary.

∽ The Right Blush for Your Complexion

Fair Skin: Blush should be a fair, light pink. Pale pinks or peach tones will brighten the inner pink tones already in your complexion.

Olive Skin: Pick an orangey-pink blush that highlights the natural "flush" tones olive skin has. You can also mix a pink blush and bronzer.

Tan Skin: Try blushes in golden pink (almost orange looking). It will complement the yellow undertones already found. But don't use anything too orange ... think of a lighter shade like peach.

Dark Skin: Blushes that are too light won't look natural, so pick rich berry colors like plum, deep purples, and deep pinks.

ꙮ BEAUTY CONFIDENTIAL: Best Left to the Professionals

My first real beauty experience came when I was in first grade, as a six-year-old living in San Diego, California. I loved to sing and convinced my mother to allow me to audition for a children's traveling singing group called Star Spangled Kids. It was small-time stuff—state fairs, mostly—but to me, it was the height of glamour and stardom.

The day of my audition, I was petrified—not because I worried about my singing abilities, but because I wasn't sure if I *looked* the part of a glamorous traveling singer. (Even at that tender age, I realized that first impressions were key.) There wasn't much I could do with my shoulder-length, wheat-colored, blunt-cut hair, and I thought wearing eye shadow would be overkill. But what about blush? *Wouldn't that make my cheeks look all pretty and make me look really special?* I thought. I surreptitiously rummaged around in my mother's makeup bag, stealing one of her blush compacts and applying it on the school bus. The audition wasn't until after school, but, hey—why not look super-glam all day long? I didn't actually know *how* to apply blush, but surely it couldn't be that hard. I glopped it on.

Who Knew?

The word "makeup" was actually coined by Max Factor.

An hour into the school day, I was summoned to the nurse's office. "Are you feeling okay, sweetheart?" she asked me, concerned. "Your teacher sent you here because she thinks you might be sick or have some kind of heat rash." She peered at me. "Your entire face is red as a tomato." I suddenly realized that perhaps my blush-applying abilities were not as stellar as I'd thought. Deeply mortified and humiliated, I decided that the best thing to do was agree that, yes, I was feeling *slightly* ill, but that it wasn't anything to worry about. No dice. She called my mother and I was sent home from school immediately. I missed the audition and spent that evening crying in the bathroom, embarrassed that I'd gotten it so, desperately wrong. (Luckily for me, I was able to reschedule the audition and was, mercifully, picked to join the group. I still to this day haven't fessed up to my mother about the unseemly blush incident.)

Pick up any women's magazine, turn to the table of contents, and you'll inevitably see a tiny reproduction of the cover shot, complete with details about the makeup used to create the look. What you may not realize, however, is that the products given credit are almost *never* the same ones used by the makeup artist on the shoot. While popular drugstore and department stores brands are often mentioned (only one brand per month, of course), in actuality, the makeup artist has used a wide variety of items from her own tool kit: a little Laura Mercier concealer here, a little Smashbox foundation there, a dab of Makeup Forever powder for good measure. After the cover is shot, and when the issue is going into print, the advertising department of a magazine decides which brand to feature that month—i.e., Cover Girl, Revlon, Maybelline—and then photos are scrutinized to determine which colors can be named that look similar. So, in actuality, you're not buying the makeup used on the cover model . . . you're just buying makeup that *looks* like the makeup used on the cover model. Egads! Hardly one of the great scams of our time—I mean, I don't think anybody's going to jail for claiming that it's Max Factor eyeshadow when in fact it's MAC—but helpful for you to realize when you buy the foundation hoping it'll recreate Gisele's complexion . . . only to realize it doesn't *quite* look the same on you.

∾ Picking Makeup Brushes

Most beauty experts will advise you to invest in a good quality set of makeup brushes ("Sure, they're expensive, but you'll use them so much, they'll practically pay for themselves and it makes *such* a difference in the appearance of your makeup!"), but I think this advice is often misleading. If you're photographed frequently (say you're an aspiring actress or model), a perfectionist or an absolute makeup whore, then go ahead, and yes, buy the best-quality brushes you can afford. (Shu Uemura, MAC, Bobbi Brown, and Smashbox all make excellent-quality brushes.) If, however, you're more the kind of gal who loves makeup, but spends ten or fifteen minutes—not forty-five—applying it in the morning, or if (let's be real here) you're too lazy to take care of expensive brushes properly, or you just don't have the money, or you don't *really* care, then I say forget it. Makeup artists are divided on the question, but many use their fingers on clients to apply foundation, concealer, some blushes (such as cream or liquid), and lip color. Yes, you'll need a blush brush (and—if you wear it—a powder brush, too), and no, you can't use the crappy little brushes that come in the container, as these will make your blush go on streaky and are just unfortunate for everybody involved. Sephora and L'Oreal both make inexpensive brushes that you can buy individually, and if you're curious about, say, how your foundation or eyeshadow would look applied with a brush, then you can tiptoe your way into the waters. If you find you're using and loving the brushes, *then* start buying more, and ones of better quality. Otherwise, honestly, you can leave it to the pros.

∾ Taking Care of Your Brushes

Okay, so you decided to go for the brushes. Yes, it's a bit more effort, and yes it's probably not necessary, but it certainly can make the entire makeup experience more fun and glamorous. It's important to properly take care of your brushes, however, regardless of how much they cost, because they can be a breeding ground for bacteria (gross, huh?), and won't make much of a difference in makeup application if they're caked with old product. (Obviously.) You can either purchase a brush-cleaning kit or wipes from the drugstore or department store (such as Clinique Make Up Brush Cleaner), or use gentle shampoo (such as Aveda Shampure or Johnson and Johnson No More Tears Shampoo). Rinse the brushes in water, then gently rub in a small amount of shampoo, lathering and rinsing well until the water runs clear. (You may need to lather up a few times to remove all traces of makeup residue if you haven't washed your brushes in a while.) Try to wash your brushes once a week, but if you forget (hey, you're a busy gal), make sure to do it at least once a month. Good quality brushes should last for several years—yes, making your big investment worthwhile.

CHAPTER SEVEN PRODUCT PRICE GUIDE

$: less than $10
$$: between $10 and $24
$$$: between $25 and $49
$$$$: between $50 and $100
$$$$$: more than $100

Clinique 3-Step System, $$$$, *clinique.com*
Bare Escentuals i.d. bareMinerals, $$$, *sephora.com*
DermaBlend, $$, *dermablend.com*
Laura Mercier Secret Camouflage, $$, *lauramercier.com*
Yves Saint Laurent Touche Éclat Radiant Touch, $$$,
 nordstrom.com
L'Oreal Paris True Match Concealer, $, drugstores
Dermablend Smooth Concealer, $$, *dermablend.com*
Smashbox Photo Finish Primer, $$$, *sephora.com*
Laura Mercier Oil-Free Foundation Primer, $$$,
 lauramercier.com
Trish McEvoy Even Skin Face Primer, $$, *trishmcevoy.com*
OC8, $$, *oc8.com*
MAC Blot, $$$, *maccosmetics.com*
Benefit Benetint, $$, *benefitcosmetics.com*
NARS Orgasm, $$, *narscosmetics.com*
Benefit Dandelion, $$$, *benefitcosmetics.com*
Smashbox O-Glow, $$$, *sephora.com*
Shu Uemura brushes, $$$, *shuuemura-usa.com*
MAC brushes, $$$, *maccosmetics.com*
Bobbi Brown, $$–$$$$, *bobbibrowncosmetics.com*

Smashbox, $$–$$$$, *smashbox.com*
Sephora brushes, $$–$$$$$, *sephora.com*
L'Oreal brushes, $, drugstore
Clinique Make Up Brush Cleaner, $$, *clinique.com*
Aveda Shampure, $$, *aveda.com*
Johnson & Johnson No More Tears Baby Shampoo, $,
   drugstores

Eight

Lips

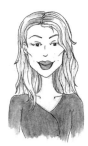

Why should Angelina Jolie have all the fun?

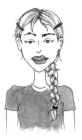

Then

Now

Once upon a time, there was a golden couple named Brad and Jen. They had golden hair, golden hearts, golden smiles. They were perfect . . . or so it seemed. One day, a tempting lass named Angie came along and stole our brave hero right out from under Jen's nose. People wept. Volcanoes erupted. Countries plunged into war. Those were dark days indeed. Why did Prince Brad succumb to fair Angelina's charms? Was it her noble spirit? Her cascading mane? Her wee babes? I am convinced I know the answer. It was, in fact, her lips.

Women with full, luscious lips are always going on about how they were teased mercilessly as children, nicknames like "Ducky" haunting their dreams. Of course, the so-called ugly duckling inevitably blossoms into a swan (Do kids not read fairy tales anymore? Don't they *know* this?), and the lips that were once a curse suddenly become a blessing. This allows the rest of us to roll our eyes and shake our fists at the gods when supermodels moan that they *used* to feel ugly.

What is it about full lips that drives men to distraction and sends so many women straight to the dermatologist, seeking to plump themselves up with collagen? As with many desired beauty traits, the roots are in biology. Scientific research shows that women with higher levels of estrogen also typically have fuller lips. (Nonscientific research, such as, you know, when you're out at a bar staring down other women who are sexier and attracting more men than you, confirms it.) So, in fact, full lips are a way for women to signal to men that their fertility is high, thereby attracting men who are desperate for babies.

And there you have it. I've solved the mystery.

Not born with lips like Angelina Jolie, Denise Richards, or Jessica Biel? It *is* possible to maximize your pout. According to a *Glamour* article, women spent $1.6 billion (biiillion!) on lip injectables like Restylane, Hylaform, and collagen in 2006, a figure that will likely be three times as high by 2010. If that sausage-like, wasp-stung look isn't what you're after, however, there *are* actually other ways to plump your pucker.

∾ Lip Plumpers

I know what you're thinking, "Yeah, *right*, some tube of gloss is going to inflate my lips." Believe it or not, however, there are several glosses and balms available that will do just that. The key ingredient is a hexapeptide called Maxi-Lip, which stimulates collagen—up to 350% with regular use!—and helps lips grow thicker and firmer, reducing and smoothing wrinkles. After just a week of using products with Maxi-Lip, you'll see an increase in collagen and a noticeably larger pout; after four weeks, your lip volume can increase up to 146%, with a 39% decrease in the depth of wrinkles. (It's important to point out, however, that you must use the Maxi-Lip products two or three times a day, every single day. It may sound gimmicky, but once you stop using the products, the effects will slowly decrease.) Of course, you could always just elect to only leave the house during your period—believe it or not, your lips are actually fuller then, thanks to increased estrogen levels. Who knew?

∾ The List: Best Lip Plumpers

Fusion Beauty LipFusion XL: A combination of micro-collagen and moisture-attracting hyaluronic acid makes this the queen of lip inflators. Apply at night for maximum benefits, or just slick on dry, clean lips during the day for a pillowy, glossy look.

City Lips Lip Plumper: With super peptide MaxiLip, the more you use this all-star, the larger your pucker will become.

Du-Wop Lip Venom: One of the original plumpers, this product relies on cinnamon and ginger to temporarily enlarge lips while also providing a tingly feeling that many women have become addicted to. Careful—it's not for the faint of heart (or lip)!

∿ Red Lips: To Go There, or Not to Go There?

The only thing sexier than full, luscious lips? A rosy-red, old Hollywood-style pucker. Red lipstick, typically associated with sexpot femme-fatales, isn't for everybody. Number one, because it draws attention to your lips, it's not the best look for women whose pouts are already big. (Have you seen photos of Angelina Jolie with cherry-red lips? It's overkill.) Number two, if you're the lazy type, forget it. You can still get rosy lips with red-tinted glosses or lip stains, but the whole process of applying, lining, blotting, and reapplying—not to mention discreetly checking your makeup compact every five minutes to make sure none has migrated on your teeth—is just too much work. Trust me. And another consideration is the fact that many guys like red lipstick in theory, but not so much when it's on a girl they're about to (or hope to) kiss. If you *are* willing to put in the time and effort, here are some tricks to ensure the lipstick stays on your lips—and doesn't end up, say, on his cheek.

∿ How To: Apply Red Lipstick

▶ Prep your lips with a light layer of foundation. This will minimize both the outline of your lips—allowing you to "create" the lip wherever you want—and the chances of the lipstick bleeding all over your face, Courtney Love–style.

▶ Dust powder lightly on lips, to help the color stick.

▶ Choose a lipliner in the same color as your lipstick, and carefully line lips, taking care not to draw too far outside the lipline.

▶ Blot lips using a tissue.

▶ Use lip brush to apply a matching color to your lips, beginning at the center of your lips and then working outward. Avoid a fake, cakey look by going easy on the color.

✑ Tips for Wearing Red

▶ Keep the rest of your makeup at least semi-natural looking. While, nowadays, red lipstick is a "go anywhere" look, red lipstick plus flushy-blush and super-dramatic eye makeup just screams "go anywhere . . . for a thousand dollars." Not quite what you're after.

▶ Try bronzer instead of blush. It will add color to your face without being overkill.

▶ If you're going to a dressy event where you're trying to channel old-time film sirens (instead of, say, pulling a Gwen and heading to the gym), make sure the rest of your look is polished—manicured nails, well-groomed brows, and thin liquid or kohl eyeliner.

∾ Celebs Who've Got the Red Lipstick Thing Down

What's more glamorous and old-Hollywood than fire-engine red, Marilyn Monroe–style lips? There's a fine line, however, between goddess, and little girl playing with Mommy's makeup—or, worse, Bozo the Clown. Take a page from these celebrities who rock red lipstick like they were born with a crimson pout.

Who Knew?

1,484 tubes of lipstick are sold every minute in the U.S.A.

Gwen Stefani: When was the last time you saw a photo of Gwen without her trademark red lips? Even while nine months pregnant and ready to burst, or just a few weeks after giving birth, Miss Stefani rarely ventured out in public without her brazen lips. Gwen makes the red-lipped look, traditionally associated with haughty evening glamour, modern by often pairing it with casual clothing, like tracksuits and tank tops.

Pink: While Pink is anything but girlie, the rocker often shows her feminine side with bold, crimson lips, mixing punk and princess with panache. Proof that you don't have to be a beauty-pageant queen to pull off look-at-me lips.

Scarlett Johansson: This is a girl who's got the beauty thing down. Despite being barely out of her teens, Scarlett has been rockin' the red lipstick for years, showing that even younger girls can wear red without looking grandmotherly.

Who Knew?

Leonardo DaVinci
reportedly spent
twelve years
painting the lips
of the Mona Lisa.

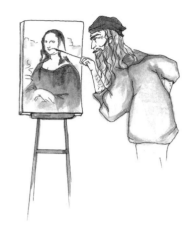

∾ On Your Lips, Not Your Glass

A great trick to keep any kind of lip color from migrating: discreetly run your tongue over your teeth and on the edge of your glass. I don't know how, I don't know why, but the saliva keeps color from sticking. Another tip: before going out, carefully put your finger in your mouth and then slide it out, and then gently blot your finger under the very bottom of your lower lip, where it meets your skin. This will pick up any stray color on the insides of your lips that could soon find its way to your teeth, and will also help keep color from slopping up your chin if you smile or take a bite of food.

The Best Color for You

Finding the right lipstick shade is all about matching it to your skin tone. A contrasting color will look harsh, garish, or simply *wrong*, whereas the right one will brighten up your complexion, and likely make your teeth look whiter, too. If you've always said, "I'm just one of those girls who can *only* wear mauve," or "I absolutely *can't* wear red," then you've probably just been choosing the wrong colors!

Picking the Right Red

OKAY, SO HOW CAN I TELL IF I'M WARM OR COOL?

It seems so retro to focus on whether you have a "warm" or a "cool" complexion, but it truly is helpful when trying to figure out what shades of lipstick will work best on you. (It's helpful, in fact, across the makeup board, but lipstick is one of those immediate, visceral things that, when it looks wrong, you feel the need to correct *immediately*. You leave the house wearing the wrong shade of eyeshadow . . . eh. Whatever. Wrong shade of lipstick? You'll be in the bathroom eighteen seconds later rubbing your pout raw to get off every last trace of color. And you know you will, too.) To get yourself pointed in the right direction, consider your heritage. Are you Scandinavian, English, Scottish, or Irish? You're probably cool. Italian, French, Black, Greek, Asian, or Middle-Eastern? You're likely warm. While warmer complexions tan easily and will usually be golden brown by the end of the summer, cool skin is often pale, burns easily, and tends to have ruddiness. If your skin is a classic English rose complexion (cool) you will easily be able to wear most reds. The rose tone of your skin will be perfectly complimented by a true red or a more pink red.

If you're cool: Choose lipsticks that also have a bluish tinge, and stay away from ones with orangey undertones. You should be able to wear true reds and pinkish reds, as well as light pinks and deep berry, wine-colored, or crimson shades.

If you're warm: For those with a more golden or olive complexion, the exact opposite will apply. Orange-y reds, such as tomato or brick, will look wonderful and true reds will also look great. Avoid cool reds with blue undertones, and stay away from pinkie reds at all costs.

A Quick Cheat-Sheet

If you're pale with blue undertones (cool) . . .
choose a pinkish red or deep reds with blue undertones.

If you have a light, ruddy, reddish
complexion (warm) . . .
choose an orange-red.

If you have golden skin and tan easily (warm) . . .
choose an orange-red.

If your skin is olive skin/slightly yellowish (warm) . . .
choose a peachy, coral, or orange-red.

∾ Moving Makeup Into the Twenty-first Century

Now, I know just a few paragraphs ago I warned against pairing deep red lipstick with heavy, dramatic eyes. This rule generally holds true. However, this doesn't mean that, when you're rocking a smoky eye, you can't wear any lipstick at *all*. Rather, go for a shade that's less attention-grabbing than red, perhaps a plum, or mauve, or glossy pink. Conversely, when your lips are the focus on your face, you don't need to have undead, Gwyneth Paltrow-without-any-makeup eyes. (Like mine, alas!) Light browns, taupe, pale gray, or muted violet could all work nicely to play up your eyes without stealing attention from your lips. In general, if you look in the mirror and think, "Wait . . . do I have too much makeup on?", you probably do. Simply rub off a little eye shadow (or blot your too-bright lip-stick and apply a paler tone), and you'll likely be good to go.

> **TIP:** *Red lipstick tends to bleed more than any other lipcolor. My favorite way of stopping that is to use* DuWop's Reverse Lipliner. *It works as a frame to keep your lipstick in place. Apply it first, and then apply lip color.*
>
> **Shalini Vadhera,**
> **celebrity makeup artist and**
> **author of *Passport to Beauty***

∾ Is Lip Balm Addictive?

When I was in high school, my best friend A.'s boyfriend J. was obsessed with Carmex. He would carry that distinctive little yellow-black-and-white tin in his pocket and 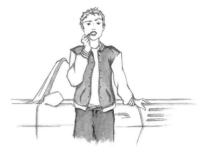 apply it—over and over and over and over—throughout the day. I thought it was kind of weird, not to mention noticed that it always made his lips look pink and shiny, sort of similar to those of our homecoming queen. Then I went off to college, and forgot all about J., and his pink, shiny lips, and his Carmex addiction. At some point in my college career, however (why cannot I remember? Why?), I, too, fell victim to the lip balm trap. My poison was not Carmex, however—which, although I cannot actually *prove*, I am certain does not contain fiberglass, as is popularly rumored—but instead Kiehl's Lip Balm # 1. My problem likely started off slowly, as do most, steadily increasing to a preoccupation, then a dependence, then a full-blown addiction. I cannot see without my contacts or eyeglasses (I mean, we're talking colors and shapes here). I cannot step out in the sun for two minutes without getting red and freckly (it's very sexy), and I am terrified of prematurely aging. Yet, were I in the bizarre position of ever being *forced* to pick one item to take with me to a deserted island—if I were, say, on *Survivor*—I would not even hesitate in taking along my trusty lip balm. (I actually sleep with one under my pillow, for the love of God, just in case I wake up in the middle of the night in a chapped-lipped panic.) It is a true problem. Damn you, lip balm makers of the world, for exposing me to this wonderful curse. Damn you.

Okay, that's all well and good and dramatic, but is it actually *addictive*? According to scientists, the answer is no . . . and yes. When you repeatedly add so much moisture to your lips, you can stunt your natural moisture-producing capabilities. So your lips, which are used to having a layer of hydration, but are now less able to produce it on their own, may need a little artificial help. Add in the fact that many lip balms contain irritating menthol or camphor, which can actually dry out your lips, and it's no wonder that you're reaching for the balm every few hours!

> **Who Knew?**
>
> *The average woman consumes four to nine pounds of lipstick in her lifetime.*

As a lip balm addict myself, I don't have the answer for you. Try to stay away from medicated lip balms, which are best used only when necessary (such as if you have a cold sore), and look for long-lasting or widely praised ones. Below, my personal favorites.

Kiehl's Lip Balm # 1: Insanely goopy (but in a good . . . nay, fabulous . . . way), this balm will stick to your lips like glue and keep them moisturized for hours. One of my all-time favorite, must-have products.

ChapStick: The classic standby, good not only because it comes in seemingly endless tasty flavors, but also because when you're in a pinch and have left your lip balm at home and absolutely, positively need one *right now*, you're bound to find one on any corner in America. Great for when you want just a thin layer of hydration.

Burt's Bees Beeswax Lip Balm: With a buttery, soft consistency, this balm (Burt's Bees' number one product) slides onto lips so smoothly that you'll find yourself reaching for it all day long.

Chapter Eight Product Price Guide

$: less than $10
$$: between $10 and $24
$$$: between $25 and $49
$$$$: between $50 and $100
$$$$$: more than $100

Fusion Beauty LipFusion XL, *sephora.com*
City Lips Lip Plumper, $$, *sephora.com*
DuWop Lip Venom, $$, *sephora.com*
DuWop Reverse LipLiner, $$, *sephora.com*
Carmex, $, drugstores
Kiehl's Lip Balm # 1, $, *kiehls.com*
ChapStick, $, drugstores
Burt's Bees Beeswax Lip Balm, $, *burtsbees.com*

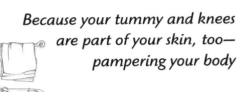

Nine

Body

*Because your tummy and knees
are part of your skin, too—
pampering your body*

For many people, a massage is a luxurious, indulgent treat—
something that only happens a few times a year, if you're
lucky. For a beauty editor, it's a regular occurrence: once a
month? Every other week? Who can keep track, what with all
the press trips and spa openings thrown into the deal? Beauty
editors become massage experts, able to tell you the difference
between shiatsu, Swedish, Reiki, hot stone, and Thai. It's all
part of the bargain. Not bad, huh? I can't remember my first
massage, but I can remember my best: a three-hour massage
journey at the sublime Clairmont Resort and Spa in Berkeley,
California, that began with a twenty-minute soak in a private,
rose-petal-filled tub overlooking the bay, then followed with an
hour-long natural-ingredient scrub (think lots of ground-up

nuts and brown sugar) in a softly lit personal shower room, followed by a quick nap on a sunken massage table with wraps swaddling my body to allow the scrub-and-oil ingredients to penetrate and hydrate the skin, and finally culminating in an out-of-this world sonic massage in yet *another* room where aromatic oils were massaged all over my pampered little body as special bowls were placed and rung on my various chakras to create vibrations to soothe and heal. By the end, I was not only passed out asleep, but also drooling. (Literally.)

Yep. All in a day's work.

The massages are killer, to be sure, but what's almost better is the use of the beauty closet as your own personal Sephora, to be browsed and ransacked both to bring home products to try for yourself, and also to gift to "needy" friends and family members. (Trust me, this comes in *really* handy at Christmas and birthdays.) Most beauty closets have an abundance of makeup, skin care, hair tools and serums, but, for me, the most fabulous thing about being an editor is the embarrassing amount of indulgent, lushly fragrant, maybe-you-don't-need-them-but-they're-still-*so*-divine-that-you-can't-resist perfumes, body soaks, and candles.

Okay, I'll admit it. I'm something of a whore for scented

> The most common error made in matters of appearance is the belief that one should disdain the superficial and let the true beauty of one's soul shine through. If there are places on your body where this is a possibility, you are not attractive—you are leaking.
>
> *Fran Lebowitz*

things. A year into my first job, I had between thirty and forty perfumes cluttering up my vanity, some of which I'd only sprayed on myself once or twice. But how can you resist when you have an entire world of Chanel, Hermès, Creed, Guerlain, Givenchy, and Jo Malone at your disposal? If *you* could, you're a much better woman than I. As a result, I'm something of an expert on yummy, froufrou things that you don't actually need. In a way, that's all beauty products really are: indulgent, gorgeous, happiness-inducing luxuries that help take you away from your reality and transport you to another world, one where you're always beautiful, always feeling your best, and always smelling divine.

∽ Turning Your Bathroom into an At-Home Spa

Sometimes (well, okay, often times), it can be fun to embrace your inner Elle Woods and be as *girly* as possible. Just because your tub is generously lined with luxurious body creams, designer bath salts, and overly fragrant shower gels in the age of postmodern feminism doesn't make you a bad person, right? For some people, it's all about the Dove soap (still classic after all these years!), but for others, nothing less than a lavender-rose-plum foaming body smoothie is going to cut it . . . and that's okay, too. At-home spa pampering has been on the rise the past few years, and it's a trend that I embrace wholeheartedly. (In theory, of course, since I am usually too lazy to do said self-pampering more than once a year. Hey,

I'm being honest here.) Turning your bathroom into a Bliss outpost is easier than you may think—yes, even you soap-and-water chicks who don't know what the hell the difference is between an exfoliator and sugar scrub and are still using those icky, bacteria-breeding poofs you can buy at the drugstore. (I say this with love and totally without judgment.)

YOUR BATH CHECKLIST

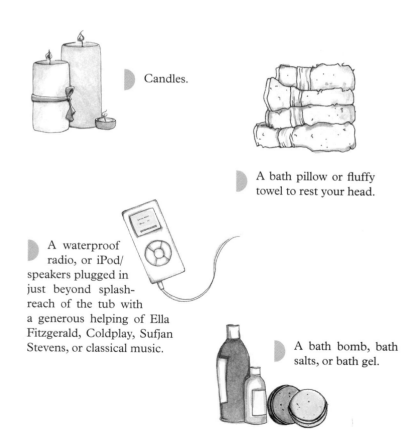

Candles.

A bath pillow or fluffy towel to rest your head.

A waterproof radio, or iPod/ speakers plugged in just beyond splash-reach of the tub with a generous helping of Ella Fitzgerald, Coldplay, Sufjan Stevens, or classical music.

A bath bomb, bath salts, or bath gel.

▶ Fragrant shower gel (preferably in the same scent as your favorite perfume and/or body lotion).

▶ In-shower body lotion or body lotion for when you step out of the shower.

▶ Exfoliating body wash, a sugar scrub, or a salt scrub.

▶ A waterproof, hanging shower radio (so you can belt out Christina Aguilera and pretend that the neighbors and/or your man can't hear you).

∾ The List: Best Indulgent Bath and Body Products

Benefit Bathina body lotion: How do I explain the amazing scent of this rich body lotion? Picture a newborn who's just had a bath and smells clean and fresh and baby-like, and then has been hugged by an angel, who happens to be wearing the most subtle, wonderful, powdery, soft fragrance in the world. And then bottle it. And then you have Bathina.

Hermès Eau d'Orange Verte Orange Givree Freshness Wake Up Gel: While the orange-with-a-hint-of-manly-leather scent is not going to be everybody's cup of tea, the fact remains that this is quite possibly the most glamorous shower gel ever created. I mean, it's *Hermès*. Do I even need to explain further? (As you can guess from the above description, it's obviously unisex, so hide it from your significant other, especially if he's a metrosexual-type. He will love it; you will weep when it's gone.)

Lush bath bombs: It's hard to choose just one product from the glorious natural, handmade confections that come out of Lush's factories, but I'm going to go with the bath bombs for their sheer cuteness and fun factor. Drop one in the bath, watch it fizz, inhale as your bathroom suddenly smells like a garden. (My personal favorite is the green Avobath bomb.)

Fresh Brown Sugar Body Polish: The original, the classic, the best sugar scrub ever. Scoop a generous handful of this scrub-and-oil concoction out of its tub while in the shower and slather all over your body until your skin is pink and glowy and exfoliated. Best of all, the oil leaves a slight layer of yummy, brown sugar-y fragrance on your skin, which means you don't even have to moisturize after.

Jo Malone Lime, Basil, and Mandarin Shower Gel: Of all the delicious Jo Malone flavors, this is both the most unisex (good or bad, depending on how you and the I-promise-you-that-he-will-become-addicted man in your life look at it) and the most classic. No matter how you slice Jo's signature fragrance, you'll love.

∽ BEAUTY CONFIDENTIAL: The Press Trip (AKA: An Excuse to Have Five Massages in Four Days)

You know what would be really fun? If you got to go to Las Vegas or Iceland for five days on a private jet and stay at a ritzy hotel and meet celebrities and dine at the finest restaurants and write an article afterward and call it "work." Hey! Wait! That's what beauty editors get to do! It's called a press trip . . . and it's fabulous. Of course, I'm being silly—press trips really *are* work, the same way that food editors get to 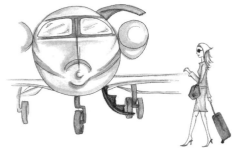 (oops, I mean "have to") go to fancy-schmancy eateries and get treated like the second coming of Henry VIII so you can know which ones are worth blowing your hard-earned cash on. There's not very much sleep, lots of not-always-fun schmoozing with various executives and publicists, copious note-taking, and so many presentations on soon-to-be-released products that you'd be happy never to hear the words "peptide" and "your readers" ever again. But let's call a spade a spade. Anything that involves a generous amount of aromatherapy, deep-tissue massages, and pedicures is never going to be difficult. Unless, of course, you're the type of person who feels weird about a stranger rubbing their hands all over your body, especially when you're lying on your back with only a towel covering your chest, and feeling hands coming uncomfortably close to . . . ahh, watch it there! Oh, of course, it's her job. Okay, where were we? That's right, having a massage and calling it work. Yeah, it's tough. Seriously.

∾ The Joy of Perfume

Sure, we all wore stuff from The
Body Shop and Bath and Body Works
when in elementary school and middle school. (And, in fact, I still love
browsing through these stores.) But
with classic, "adult" perfume, I started young. My father took a business

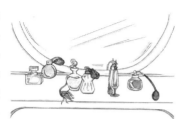

trip to France when I was thirteen, and brought back a bottle
of Guerlain Shalimar, the first oriental fragrance that famously scandalized the world when it was created and remains an
iconic bestseller to this day. It only took one spritz to hook me,
since it conjured up images of Paris and romance and mystery (the kind that women who were sixteen years old were
obviously having daily). I sprayed Shalimar on my wrists and
neck, and set off into my little world, secure in the knowledge
that I smelled glamorous, grown-up, delicious. My friends, by
contrast, only had one thing to say: "Um . . . you smell like
my grandma." It's kind of disconcerting to have your friends
wrinkle their noses everytime you walk into a room, but the
nose likes what it likes. I continued wearing Shalimar and still
wear it to this day. Except for when I cheat on it with other perfumes . . . which is basically daily. Call me a fragrance
commitment-phobe.

Just as people are finally bending the rules when it comes
to wine ("Only white with fish! Only red with meat!"), we've
now made our way into the crazy future of perfume, where
it's not only permissible but encouraged to have a scent ward-

robe. Why limit yourself to one perfume when you can have sixteen? Or, well, at least three. After all, you wouldn't wear the same shoes everyday, would you?

A QUICK FRAGRANCE PRIMER

Perfume should be easy—spritz it on, smell delicious!—but it's often difficult to find the one fragrance (or seven) that screams *you* and works with your unique body chemistry. By learning the various fragrance terms, you can maximize your chances of finding a great scent. Perfumers divide fragrance up into several different categories, but for your purposes, I've combined a few.

Floral: This one is a no-brainer. It smells like flowers. Popular ingredients include night-blooming jasmine—sounds silly, but because its petals open at night, jasmine is often picked then, when its scent is strongest—gardenia, magnolia, and rose.

Oriental: Usually describes sophisticated, spicy fragrances with notes like amber, vanilla, and musk.

Fresh: Think bright, sunny, and light-as-air. These fragrances, which can further be broken down into a few different categories, might have fruity notes such as grapefruit and mandarin, a watery, sea-breeze characteristic, or a certain crispness to them.

Green/Woody: Either slightly heavier, with cedar, woodsy, and spicy notes, or with the aroma of a wet garden. Think pine, moss, patchouli, and sandalwood, combined with citrus and a touch of fruit. These scents are often more popular in men's fragrance.

Perfume . . . cologne . . . eau de toilette . . . it's all the same, right? Well, no, not really. Perfume extract is the costliest form of fragrance, with the highest percentage of essential oils (typically around 25%), followed by eau de parfum, which is about 15% to 20% oil. Eau de toilette follows with around 10% or 15% oil, then eau de cologne (3% or 4%), and finally the super-light eau fraiche (just 1% or 2%). Most of what you'll find at the drug or department store will be eau de parfum or eau de toilette, and it's up to you to decide how much you want to spend, since eau de parfum is always more expensive—of course, the higher the percentage of essential oils, the more it'll cost you. But who wants to put a price on smelling nice? All in the name of beauty.

TIP: *When testing out fragrances, try no more than three at a time, and give them an hour to develop—walk around the mall, do some shopping, or come back the next day. What you don't like at first sniff might develop, twenty minutes later, into your all-time favorite scent; it happens all the time.*

MODERN PERFUMES THAT ARE ALREADY CLASSICS

Angel by Thierry Mugler: One of the most popular, innovative scents of all time, Angel is polarizing—either you *love* it or you *hate* it. With notes of chocolate, vanilla, honey, and caramel, it's utterly mouthwatering, but definitely not for the faint of heart. Best not to wear in close quarters, or on a first date—unless you know for sure that he won't run screaming in the other direction (or you just don't give a damn).

Chanel Coco Mademoiselle: Inspired by the runaway success of the more heavily amber Chanel Coco, this fresh oriental contains bright orange and bergamot combined with musky patchouli and vetiver for an unexpected combination that's sweet and sexy at the same time.

Narciso Rodriguez for Her: As musky and mysterious as they come, with amber, honey flower, and woody notes. Sophisticated enough to wear to the office, sexy enough to wear to the lounge, and sensual enough to wear with nothing at all. Has a fantastic drydown and clings to your wrists for hours. One of my all-time favorites, this is the perfume I reach for more than any other.

Stella by Stella McCartney: A classic rose scent, but made unexpected and modern thanks to its mix of fresh, bracing mandarin and sensual amber. You'll find it on every fashion diva's vanity.

Eau de Issey by Issey Miyake: A runaway bestseller in the 90s and one of the first marine fragrances, this is light, crisp, and has a faint lemony scent. The antithesis of the heavy 80s fragrances, and good for women who simply want to smell natural and pretty, not perfumey.

Dolce and Gabbana Light Blue: Feminine and fresh, with lemon, apple, jasmine, and base notes of cedarwood and musk.

Bulgari Eau de Thé Verte: It's exactly what it sounds like:

green tea, but with no tartness, only a sweet aroma. Started the green tea scent craze.

Marc Jacobs: Not for wallflowers, the strong, clear gardenia, and wild muguet notes make themselves noticed the second you walk into a room. While it seems like one of those scents that's going to wear you, it quickly mingles with your chemistry, and after a few hours, smells different on everybody.

CLASSIC PERFUMES THAT ARE STILL MODERN

Creed Fleurissimo: The famed fragrance house, which has been around for centuries and often did commissions for royals, created this perfume for Princess Grace on her wedding day. Over fifty years later, it still holds up to scrutiny—floral, floral, floral.

Chanel Number 5: Not everybody's cup of tea (okay, I'll admit that I can't stand it), but you can't have a fragrance list without this purposely-chemical-smelling juggernaut, right? Marilyn Monroe famously claimed that she wore two drops of it to bed, and nothing else.

Who Knew?

According to Chanel, a bottle of No. 5 is sold every thirty seconds.

Guerlain Shalimar: The original oriental fragrance, with heavy vanilla and bergamot, just a tiny bit goes a long way. Reportedly inspired by the Indian emperor Shah Jahangir, who built the Taj Mahal for his wife after her death.

Hermès Eau d'Orange Verte: Unisex, with lemon and mandarin orange, papaya, mango, and patchouli, this sprays on sharp, but dries down quietly, lingering on skin longer than many other citrus-based scents. Best worn with a Barbour coat and Wellies.

Tresor by Lancôme: With rose, muguet, lilac, and apricot blossom, this is one of those lovely, classic, delightful fragrances that will never go out of style, simply because it smells so damn wonderful.

L'Air du Temps by Nina Ricci: Created in the late 40s, L'Air du Temps's soft rosewood, neroli, peach, and vetiver still smells fresh and romantic—not anachronistic—today.

Opium by Yves Saint Laurent: An incredibly exotic fragrance introduced in the late 70s and stemming from Yves Saint Laurent's own fascination with the East. The top notes are floral (rose and carnation), but the scent is brimming with spices such as clove and pepper, and musky sandalwood. Wear it with a sense of irony and some "don't mess with me" boots.

IF YOU LIKE THIS ONE, TRY THAT

This is my completely unscientific, admittedly-never-trained-in-Grasse-France analysis of what scents seem to be similar to others. Based on my own (obsessive) trial and error, as well as conversations with friends and many, many wasted afternoons at Sephora, I've come up with these fragrance pairings. These scents all have similar undertones and notes, so if you particularly like one of the scents in the group, check out the others. Note that I'm making up some of the categories here (as far as I know, there isn't *actually* a scent category called "dark"), but I think they're more helpful and intuitive than typical classifications.

Fresh, soapy skin (you may also like watery, fruity, and lemon or tea scents): Sarah Jessica Parker Lovely, J. Lo Glow, Clean by D'Lish, Benefit Maybe Baby, Chanel No. 5, Bond No. 9 West Side.

Watery (you may also like fresh, soapy skin scents): Issey Miyake Eau d'Issey, Dolce and Gabbana Light Blue, Guerlain Shalimar Light.

Heavy, amber-musk (you may also like dark scents): Chanel Coco Mademoiselle, Chanel Allure Sensualle, Narciso Rodriguez for Her, Angel by Thierry Mugler, Kiehl's Original Musk Oil, Britney Spears Fantasy, Guerlain Shalimar, Givenchy Pi, Bulgari Omnia.

Fruity (you may also like lemon or tea, as well as soft florals): Ralph by Ralph Lauren, Miss Dior, Clinique Happy, Donna Karan Be Delicious, Bond No. 9 Chinatown.

Lemon or Tea (you may also like rose scents or watery scents): Annick Goutal Eau d'Hadrian, Bulgari Eau de Parfumee Green Tea, Elizabeth Arden Green Tea.

Soft florals (you may also like rose scents): Ralph Lauren Romance, Creed Spring Water, Blush by Marc Jacobs, Victoria's Secret Very Sexy for Her.

Rose (you may also like soft florals or gardenia scents): Stella McCartney Stella, Nanette Lepore, Jo Malone Red Roses.

Gardenia (you may also like heavy florals or rose scents): Michael Kors, Marc Jacobs, Kai, Chanel Gardenia.

Heavy florals (you may also like gardenia and rose scents): Calvin Klein Eternity Romance, Creed Fleurissimo, Creed

Jasmal, Fracas, Vera Wang, Guerlain Mitsouko, Editions de Parfums Frédéric Malle Lys Mediterranée.

Dark (you may also like heavy, amber-musk scents): Donna Karan Black Cashmere, YSL Nu, Dior Addict, Chanel No. 19.

How To: Make Your Perfume Last Longer

It's all about scent layering. The higher the alcohol content, the faster it will evaporate, as it's the oils in the fragrance that cling to the skin and make it envelop you in a cocoon of scent (doesn't that sound delish?) all day. To keep a nice scent lingering on you, begin in the shower with a fragrant body wash (in the same version as your perfume, if it's sold, or in a similar scent family, such as musky or floral), then apply scented lotion to damp skin after you exit the shower and pat (not rub!) yourself dry. Spritz perfume on your pulse points, such as your wrists, behind your knees, or at your neck. Many perfumes now come in oil versions, which will last longer than traditional sprays. And, of course, as we've already covered, perfume extract lasts the longest, followed by eau de parfum, then eau de toilette, and finally cologne. (I like to spray a little perfume at the base of my hair, to allow the strands to soak up a tiny bit of the oil, although this is not something that pleases my hairdresser, as the alcohol in perfume will dry out hair. Eh. I still think it's worth it.)

～ Why It's So Important to Moisturize and Wear Sunscreen (Yes, on Your Body, Too!) Every Day

You've heard ad nauseum how important it is to wear sunscreen on your face, but you may not realize that sunscreen on your body is equally important to keep skin soft, young-looking, and even toned. The best (other) places to apply sunscreen everyday? Your hands, neck, and décolleté (that's your cleavage, gals), which all start to show the sun's damaging effects very quickly. You know liver spots, those dark marks that elderly people often get on their hands? It's sun damage. Since the skin on your hands and 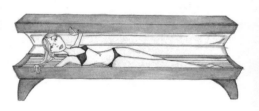 chest is thin, those areas will start to shrivel and discolor in the sun more quickly than others, leaving you resembling a dried raisin. (Well, not really, but I thought I'd try and put a little bit of fear in you. Sun is bad, folks! Baaaaaad.)

Actually, the sun is not *that* bad—yes, it does produce vitamin D, which our bodies all need, it helps regulate our internal clocks and keep us cheerful, and, of course, it feels so nice and yummy when you're lying out in your bikini. But, unfortunately, the more sun you get, the more quickly you will age, not to mention up your risk of skin cancer.

I'll confess that I've been a tanning addict on a few occasions in my life. I just feel *better* when I'm tan. However, I also feel better when my skin is clear and pretty, and too much sun, even when carefully "regulated" (just half an hour won't hurt, right?), soon brings out these nasty spots, bumps, and discolorations that I would rather avoid, thank you very much. It all comes back to vanity—my motivation is simply that I want to look twenty-seven when I'm forty. (So now, I'm a self-tanning addict and am constantly on the hunt for products that don't smell and won't turn you orange—but that's another story.)

If you're fair, with blue eyes and a Northern European background, you're of course more likely to burn than, say, somebody from Kenya. If you have a darker complexion, you aren't immune to sun damage, although you do suffer from skin cancer less often than those with fairer complexions.

The moral of the story? Tan if you must (hey, it's your skin and your life), but do realize that, eventually, it *will* catch up with you. (Have I sufficiently shamed you? Okay, good.) The real moral: don't forget the sunscreen on your body!

∽ Moisturizing and Exfoliating Advances for Lazy People

Okay, so you've dragged your ass to the shower for two days in a row (maybe, if the people around you are really lucky, every single day this week!). And now that you're out of the shower, naked, freezing and late for work, you're expected to take the time to slather cream all over your body, whistling a happy tune while birds chirp and the sun shines and you do your diva thing? Am I the only one who finds this wholly unrealistic? Sure, to some people, moisturizing after you get out of the shower is as natural as brushing your teeth after meals or washing your face before bed . . . but I often just can't be bothered, and many women I know are the same. (With the whole shower-moisturizer one-two punch, I mean. *Obviously* we brush our teeth after we eat.) Luckily, our friendly neighborhood beauty people have been slaving away over hot Bunsen burners, developing cool innovations to help us poor slobs keep our skin in tiptop shape while still making it to work only about five minutes late. Gotta love technology.

∽ Ingredients to Look For

Your best bet for taking care of your body without having to really think about it are products that work double-duty, such as in-shower moisturizers that you can slap on and sugar scrubs that exfoliate while leaving skin with a thin layer of hydration. Look for products with a combination of glycolic and lactic acid, which exfoliate dry skin cells while simultaneously moisturizing and softening. In the winter, when your skin will likely be parched and scaly, pick products with urea and glycerin; look for moisturizers containing exfoliating acids such as glycolic and salicylic during the summer, when your oil production will be up and you'll be more prone to breakouts on your body.

∽ The List: Great Body Products

Olay In Shower Gel: How smart is this? When you're in the shower, doing your thing, simply slather this lotion all over your body, then rinse off, and there's no need to put on moisturizer *after* you get out of the shower. (You know, when you're shivering and naked and freezing and the last thing you want to do is stand there longer—shivering, naked, and freezing while you put cold, wet lotion all over your rapidly goose-pimpling body.)

MD Skincare Alpha-Beta Body Peel: Just like the slavishly adored Alpha-Beta peel for the face, but with a different combination of acids and ingredients so it can effectively be used on the body (which needs tougher exfoliation). Not only will it help control breakouts on your chest and back, but the combination of exfoliating salicylic and glycolic acids will also help keep the skin on your neck and décolleté looking younger and firmer.

Clinique Acne Solutions Body Treatment Spray: When ugly, annoying zits start sprouting up all over your back, chest, and shoulders—whether it's from exercising, summer heat, or simply hormones—spritz on this salicylic acid spray, which quickly gets rid of breakouts and has a 360-degree mechanism that lets you spray it upside down.

Neutrogena Norwegian Formula Hand Cream: A beauty editor favorite, this rich, emollient hand cream lasts for hours (and hours and hours), hydrating and softening even the most chapped hands.

Johnson's Softlotion 24 Hour Moisture Body Lotion: With a subtle, softly fruity scent, this delicious lotion absorbs into skin quickly and lasts for hours (not quite twenty-four, but the entire day, nonetheless!).

Direct from Jolie in NYC:
Beauty Myth: Cellulite creams work.
Sorry. They don't.

I hate to break this to you. Really I do . . . but efficacious cellulite creams are one of those myths, like Santa Claus or men who prefer "natural" women. (The problem there is usually the male fantasy of "natural" versus the brutal female reality, but that's a whole 'nother story.) While there are some cellulite creams that have cult status (like Shiseido Body Creator Aromatic Firming Cream and Osmotics Lipoduction Body Perfecting Complex), all the creams really do is smooth out the appearance of the top of your skin. They can't actually make cellulite disappear and literally change the composition of your body, otherwise they'd have to be FDA regulated as drugs, not faux-miraculous, happiness-inducing (well, temporarily, at least) cosmeceuticals. That's not to say that you may not see a small, temporary difference in the appearance of your 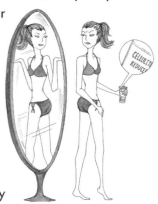 thighs and tummy after using these creams several times a day, everyday, for weeks—the same way, say, a really great foundation might make acne look like, poof! it's gone—but once you stopped using the creams, the magic would disappear. And I'm just too damn lazy to put all that time and effort into something that will probably not work, or will only provide minuscule results once it does. I haven't yet taken my own advice on this one (I mostly just stare in the mirror at my saddlebags and say, "Away! Go away!", which, alas, hasn't worked yet), but you're better off saving the time and money and just going to the gym (which won't actually make cellulite go away either, but will obviously reduce the amount of fat for the ol' cellulite to work with). And, barring that, get a really deep Mystic tan; the darker shade of skin and contours will help make it look like there's less cellulite, and aren't a great tan and thin thighs all you really need for Spring Break anyway?

∾ Nothing Makes You Look Thinner Than a Great (Fake) Tan

Okay, so we're already established that fake tans are better, at least for your skin, than real tans. The problem with fake tans? They're usually *terrible*. Even if you're a self-styled tanning expert who's been Fake Baking it for years, one misstep and you're walking around town with orange heels, streaky legs, and stained knuckles. And even on your best day, you probably still smell. (I have an ex-boyfriend who refused to get anywhere near me on days I fake-tanned, wrinkling his nose and exclaiming, "Why do you *do* that to yourself?") When done properly, however, fake tans are phenomenal—they help make you look thin and healthy, and can give limbs an alluring sheen and glow that just doesn't radiate from naked, ghost-pale skin. Most beauty editors are fake-tanned 24/7, although the past few years have seen an explosion in favor of those moisturizers with "a hint" of self-tanner.

What to look for in a self-tanner? Seek out ones with a combination of DHA and erythrulose. DHA is the standard self-tanning ingredient that helps turn you dark, but it's also the one responsible for that awful stink. Erythrulose isn't as strong-smelling, and will give your skin a hint of color without turning you orange. When their powers combine, the effect is often magic. One tanner does not fit all, so if you're fair-skinned, beware of tanners that only contain DHA, unless they come in a "light" or "fair" version. Otherwise, you're just playing with fire, Little Miss Future Oompah Loompah.

∾ How To: Self-Tan

Want to avoid those gross streaks, patchy ankles, and orange knees? Follow these steps a time or two. Soon, you'll be a self-tanning pro—and then will promptly ignore the steps, decide to improvise, and find yourself back to square one with said streaks and patches. It happens to the best of us.

1. Exfoliate in the shower with a finely-grained scrub. (Avoid oil-based scrubs that leave a moisturizing film on skin.)

2. Pat dry and moisturize with a fragrance-free, quick-absorbing lotion. (Note: lotions with shimmer, body creams, etc., etc., do not qualify, as I've learned the hard way.)

3. Wait about twenty minutes until the lotion seeps into your skin. If you don't have twenty minutes to spare, try to wait ten, or five, or two, or anything. It's not *crucial*, but it does help.

4. Decide to start from either your feet, and work your way up, or your face, and work your way down. Starting with your tummy and then spreading out in random directions will only lead to disaster and streaky patches, as you'll likely forget where you've already put tanner and then will double-apply.

5. Begin at said starting point, putting a small amount of self-tanner in your hands and working slowly in controlled, circular motions, rubbing tanner into skin well. (Note: wearing rubber gloves is completely optional. I know people who swear by it; I personally hate it and feel it ruins my self-tanning "experience." Assuming you properly remove the tanner from your hands when done, it makes little difference.)

6. Pay special attention to the tops of feet (avoid your toes, if possible), ankles, heels, knees, elbows, wrists, tops of hands (avoid your fingers and knuckles, too) and neck, which are all areas where the color will either seep in more quickly (because skin is drier there) or where mistakes will be extra-noticable.

7. If possible, enlist a friend to help you with your back. If you're not going to be in a dire situation (a photo shoot, a wedding with a backless dress, etc), then go for it yourself, contorting into your best pretzel-like positions and concentrating on the back of the shoulders, back-sides of your tummy and lower back. As long as you attempt to rub it in well and aren't using a color that's too harsh for your skintone, well, the mistakes probably won't be *too* noticeable.

8. When applying self-tanner to your face, blend well into your jawline, hairline, and ears, to avoid the "mask" of self-tanner. Avoid the area underneath your nose (too much tanner here could look like a mustache), and go easy on the chin area (ditto, but like a beard).

9. Put a dab of tanner on your index finger and apply to the top of your opposite hand, then repeat with the other hand and index finger, avoiding fingers and knuckles, and making sure all tanner is blended well at wrists.

10. Wash hands slowly and carefully, avoiding wetting your wrists or tops of hands, but taking care to get all tanner off fingers, nails, and the area in between your fingers (which is, by the way, a magnet for tanner).

And voila! Try to wait twenty minutes before you apply clothing. If not possible, wear the darkest clothing that you can find, taking care to make sure it's something you can wash or won't be torn up about if it gets tanner stains on it. Remember, white or expensive clothing and freshly applied self-tanner *do not* mix.

TIP: *If you can avoid it, don't apply the same self-tanner to your body as to your face; look for specially designed facial versions with the words "non-comedogenic" on the package to ensure you don't break out.*

Direct from Jolie in NYC:
What's wrong with real beauty?

You've surely noticed those Dove advertisements that were all over town and in magazines featuring "real" women (read: not models) in their underwear. I was fortunate enough to go on a press trip (one of the famous "private jet" trips) when Dove unveiled their Campaign for Real Beauty. Clever corporate marketing or not, it's a powerful message and all of the editors were moved by the campaign. After the presentations were finished, there wasn't a dry eye in the room; who can't relate to not feeling skinny, sexy, or pretty enough? That's why I'm surprised and kind of annoyed by some of the reactions I've heard to the ads: making fun of the big thighs, bemoaning the lack of blonds, wondering who would actually find *those* women pretty. I guess we've become so celebrity obsessed—and seduced by airbrushing—that we think if it doesn't look like Paris Hilton, Jessica Simpson, or Gisele Bundchen, it can't possibly be sexy.

Glamour magazine ran an interesting article with Aisha Tyler called "I don't want to be perfect!" where Aisha was photographed, then allowed photos of the "real" Aisha and the airbrushed Aisha placed side-by-side. Real Aisha is pretty, but airbrushed Aisha is glowy, taut, sleek, and, yes, perfect. Of course, she doesn't actually exist—but she sure is gorgeous, huh?

I think the problem with all of these ads and messages is that you have to be in the right mood and frame of mind to accept them. If you're at the gym working up a sweat on the elliptical and come across the Nike ads celebrating big butts and scraped knees and strong legs, you might think "Hell, yeah! I'm strong like that! Hear me roar!" and kick up the speed. But if you're on your way to a club, primped, powdered, lipglossed, coiffed, and dolled up to look as sexy as possible, you might pass by one of the Dove billboards and think "Thank *God* I'm skinnier than those women," and feel really pleased with yourself. (I'm guilty on that front, I'll admit it.) I guess the challenge is to get to a place where everybody sees celebrities as too skinny (because, let's be real, 95% of them are walking eating disorders) and can appreciate real women (what does that term even *mean* anymore?) in all of their real woman-ness.

∾ The List: Best Hostess Gifts

Obviously, if somebody invites you into their home for, say, a weekend visit, it's only polite to bring them a small gift in return. Flowers and wine have always been popular, but if your hostess is even remotely a beauty junkie, you might consider bringing her a small gift along the lines of candles or a home scent. Here, the best beauty hostess gifts.

Candles: The ultimate beauty gift, fabulous candles are a gorgeous addition to any home and, seeing as "designer" candles can be ridiculously expensive, are always appreciated. Look for brands like Diptyque, Red Flower, Slatkin and Co, Jo Malone, Penhaligon, or even famous designer scents in candle form, such as Marc Jacobs or Donna Karan.

Bath Gel: I'm not normally a product snob, but this only works when you splurge a bit and buy higher end bath products, such as those sold by Hermès, Jo Malone, or more democratic-but-still-chic brands like Origins or Aveda.

Home Scent: Don't worry, your hostess *probably* won't think you're trying to tell her that her home smells. Brands like Floris, Red Flower, Jo Malone, and Penhaligon all make fabulous home scents that are incredibly giftable.

∾ Candles: Not Just for Cheesy Chick-Flicks and Romantic Restaurants

Fixated on candles? You're not alone. You can find lovely candles running the price and flavor gamut, from edible scents like chocolate and mango available at drugstores, malls, and home stores to designer versions that have nuanced, rich fragrances and cost more than some accessories. Here's everything you need to know.

- Look for a lead-free wick, as this avoids getting soot on the rim and on your walls.
- Always trim the wick to one-quarter of an inch to preserve the candle.
- Never burn for more hours than recommended by the manufacturer.

CHAPTER NINE PRODUCT PRICE GUIDE

$: less than $10

$$: between $10 and $24

$$$: between $25 and $49

$$$$: between $50 and $100

$$$$$: more than $100

Products

Dove soap, $, drugstores

Benefit Bathina body lotion, $$, *benefitcosmetics.com*

**Hermès Eau d'Orange Verte Orange Givree Freshness
Wake Up Gel,** $$, *usa.Hermès.com*

Lush bath bombs, $, *lush.com*

Fresh Brown Sugar Body Polish, $$$$, *fresh.com*

Jo Malone Lime, Basil and Mandarin Shower Gel, $$$$,
jomalone.com

The Body Shop, $$, *thebodyshop.com*

Bath and Body Works, $$, *bathandbodyworks.com*

Guerlain Shalimar, $$$$, *neimanmarcus.com*

Angel by Thierry Mugler, $$$$, *saksfifthavenue.com*

Chanel Coco Mademoiselle, $$$$, *usa-chanel.com*

Narciso Rodriguez for Her, $$$$, *saksfifthavenue.com*

Stella McCartney Stella, $$$$, *neimanmarcus.com*

Issey Miyake Eau d'Issey, $$$$, *neimanmarcus.com*

Dolce and Gabbana Light Blue, $$$, *sephora.com*

Bulgari Eau de Thé Verte, $$$$, *neimanmarcus.com*

Marc Jacobs, $$$, *sephora.com*

Creed Fleurissimo, $$$$, *neimanmarcus.com*

Chanel Number 5, $$$$, *usa-chanel.com*

Hermès Eau d'Orange Verte, $$$$$, *usa-Hermès.com*

Lancôme Trésor, $$$, *lancome-usa.com*

Nina Ricci L'Air du Temps, $$$$, *sephora.com*

Yves Saint Laurent Opium, $$$$, *neimanmarcus.com*

Sarah Jessica Parker Lovely, $$$, *sarahjessicaparkerbeauty.com*

Glow by J.Lo, $$$, *shopjlo.com*

Clean by D'Lish, $$$, *sephora.com*

Benefit Maybe Baby, $$, *benefitcosmetics.com*

Bond No. 9 West Side, $$$$$, *saksfifthavenue.com*

Guerlain Shalimar Light, $$$$, *guerlain.com* for locations

Chanel Allure Sensualle, $$$$, *usa-chanel.com*

Kiehl's Original Musk Oil, $$, *kiehls.com*

Britney Spears Fantasy, $$$, *sephora.com*

Givenchy Pi, $$$$, *givenchy.com* for locations

Bulgari Omnia, $$$$, *neimanmarcus.com*

Ralph by Ralph Lauren, $$$$, *polo.com*

Miss Dior, $$$$, *eluxury.com*

Clinique Happy, $$$, *clinique.com*

Donna Karan Be Delicious, $$$, *donnakaran.com*

Bond No. 9 Chinatown, $$$$$, *saksfifthavenue.com*

Annick Goutal Eau d'Hadrian, $$$$$, *eluxury.com*

Elizabeth Arden Green Tea, $$, *elizabetharden.com*

Ralph Lauren Romance, $$$$, *polo.com*

Creed Spring Water, $$$$$, *neimanmarcus.com*

Blush by Marc Jacobs, $$$$, *marcjacobs.com*

Victoria Secret Very Sexy for Her, $$$, *victoriasecretbeauty.com*

Nanette Lepore, $$$, *neimanmarcus.com*

Jo Malone Red Roses, $$$$, *jomalone.com*

Michael Kors, $$$$, *neimanmarcus.com*

Kai, $$$, *abeautifullife.com*

Chanel Gardenia, $$$$, *usa-chanel.com*

Calvin Klein Eternity Moment, $$$$, *sephora.com*

Creed Fleurissimo, $$$$$, *neimanmarcus.com*

Creed Jasmal, $$$$$, *neimanmarcus.com*

Fracas, $$$$$, *neimanmarcus.com*

Vera Wang, $$$$, *nordstrom.com*

Guerlain Mitsouko, $$$$$, *guerlain.com* for locations

Editions de Parfums Frédéric Malle Lys Mediterranée,
$$$$$, *editionsdeparfums.com* for locations

Donna Karan Black Cashmere, $$$$, *neimanmarcus.com*

YSL Nu, $$$$, *sephora.com*

Dior Addict, $$$$, *eluxury.com*

Chanel No. 19, $$$$, *usa-chanel.com*

Olay In Shower Gel, $, drugstores

MD Skincare Alpha-Beta Body Peel, $$$$, *mdskincare.com*

Clinique Acne Solutions Body Treatment Spray, $$,
clinique.com

Neutrogena Norwegian Formula Hand Cream, $, drugstores

Johnson's Softlotion 24 Hour Moisture Body Lotion, $,
drugstores

Shiseido Body Creator Aromatic Firming Cream, $$$$,
shiseido.com

Osmotics Lipoduction Body Perfecting Complex, $$$$,
osmotics.com

Fake Bake, $$$, *fakebake.com*

Diptyque, $$$, *neimanmarcus.com*

Red Flower, $$$$, *redflower.com*

Slatkin and Co, $$$, *neimanmarcus.com*

Floris, $$$$, *florislondon.com*

Hermès, $$$$$, *usa-Hermès.com*

Origins, $$, *origins.com*
Aveda, $$, *aveda.com*
Jo Malone, $$$$, *jomalone.com*
Penhaligon, $$$$, *penhaligons.co.uk*

Spas

Claremont Resort and Spa, 41 Tunnel Road,
Berkeley, California: 510–843–3000

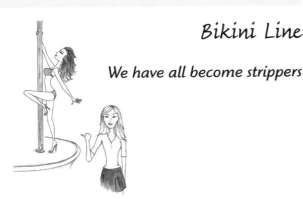

Ten

Bikini Line

We have all become strippers

Think back about, oh, seven or eight years ago. Try and remember the first time you heard about a Brazilian bikini wax. A Brazilian? you thought. Why, what's that? It sounds fun! It sounds exotic! It sounds . . . uh, wait? You mean, I'm supposed to lie spread-eagle on a table, knees smushed against my face as if I'm giving birth, naked from the waist down, in front of a complete stranger? While she drips hot wax . . . uh . . . *there*? And then rips it out of me? *There*, too? And *there*? Er . . . nevermind. Thanks, but, erm, not really my thing. I'm not a stripper.

But then all the oh-so-wholesome-looking girls in *Playboy* had them. (Well, wholesome except for that whole "naked in a magazine for the entire world, including their fathers, to see." No, *I* didn't see. But I certainly heard.) And then movie stars would giggle about them in hushed tones in "revealing"

magazine interviews (I'll say). And then Jenny, your college
roommate's cousin, got one. Your sister's best friend Sarah got
one, too. Eventually, so did *your* best friend. And they all said
it was *awesome*. Awesome? What's awesome about—okay, fine.
Just this once. Only so I can prove that it's all a fuss about
nothing.

Oh. I see. Well . . . that *is* kind of nice. It's very neat and
clean-looking. Not very womanly, though. Maybe I'll do it just
one more time. Only because it's so neat and clean. I wonder
if my boyfriend will like it?

Wow. Okay. I guess that answers *that* question. Our anniversary is coming up. I should get another one. And while I'm
there, maybe I should book an appointment for another one in
four weeks, just in case.

And then you're hooked. Suddenly, you have nether regions
identical to Bambi and Tiffani. It's a slippery slope, folks.

Just try explaining a Brazilian bikini wax to your mom. Go
on. Try. She won't get it. "But, honey, *why*? That sounds awfully painful. Do you really *like* it?" Tough question. "Well,
Mom. Do you mean, do I like the hot wax and the spread-
eagle positions and Ilsa the burly aesthetician and the painful
ripping? No. But afterwards? Um . . . *yeah*."

So it's not very feminist and women should celebrate their
natural bodies, which, us being animals and all, have hair everywhere. So it hurts like hell. So it's really, really embarrassing. But when it's your birthday or your anniversary or that all
important third date and Billy is meeting you at your house for
a candlelit dinner and you just want to look your absolute best
from head to toe and everything in between and you spent
three hours at the salon today having a mani/pedi and your
hair done—how can you not?

If you've never had a bikini wax (Brazilian or otherwise, since most waxing salons now have a full menu that rivals the selections at Per Se), you're probably scrunching your nose in disgust or confusion. If you have, you know exactly what I'm talking about. Regardless, every gal, from the novice to the most jaded waxer, feels at least a twinge of humiliation each time she climbs into that chair with those horrible paper panties. Rest assured, Ilsa has seen it all before. But to make your next time (or your first time!) as ho-hum as possible, here's everything you need to know.

∾ First Things First

EXPLORE YOUR OPTIONS

Maybe waxing just *really* isn't for you. (After a brief but passionate flirtation with it in college, I just couldn't be bothered anymore. I'm now a dedicated Venus Razor-er). Several options abound. Here, the pros and cons of the most effective and popular hair-removal methods:

Waxing: Pros are that hair grows in lighter and softer afterwards. Hair should be at least a ¼ of an inch long for the wax to stick. The con is, obviously, that it hurts. Lasts three to six weeks.

Laser: Works best on fair skin with dark hair, because melanin in skin absorbs more light. Positive factor: Lasts six months. Negative factor: Expensive. Very expensive. (We're talking approximately a thousand dollars.)

Shaving: Only lasts one to three days, but is super cheap and super quick. Can also be done in bathrooms of restaurants if it's an utter emergency. Not that I've ever gone there, but I'm just saying. (Okay, truthfully . . . I have. It *was* an utter emergency.)

⟋ Still Want the Wax? What to Expect

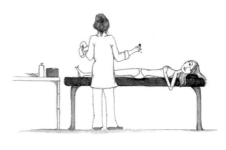

Okay, so let's just assume that you *haven't* ever been professionally waxed before. (Those of you who have, you can come along for the ride, too. Just sit back in your chairs and pat yourselves on the back that you'll never have to experience that harrowing first time again. The rest of you, please forget what I just said to those people who've been there.) It's not really *that* bad. Okay. I'm kind of lying because I don't want to scare you. But only a little bit. Here's what you can expect.

▶ Arrive at the salon to be greeted by a peppy, cheerful receptionist named Amber. She's there to soothe you and make you feel like everything's going to be all right.

▶ Get led into the private room, which usually looks something like a doctor's office, complete with raised table covered in white paper.

▶ Disrobe from the waist down. Stare at white paper panties held together by strings in disbelief. Put said piece of paper-and-strings on. Adjust at least fifteen times while lying on the table to make sure nothing is peeking out. Give up when you realize that this is impossible.

▶ Wait alone, cold, and half-naked in the room. Wonder if it's too late to put your clothes back on and flee.

▶ Say hello to Ilsa as she enters the room and immediately gets to work examining your lady-parts in-depth. Stare at the ceiling and try to make small talk as she pulls out a razor to tidy you up, then instructs you to contort into a knees-to-the-chest position that not even your boyfriend has seen. Wonder if it's too late to put your clothes back on and flee.

▶ Look at the ceiling and make small talk as she sprinkles baby powder to keep the wax from sticking.

▶ Think, "What the . . . ?" as she spreads hot wax in areas heretofore unseen by the light of day.

▶ Squeal in pain as she rips hot wax out of areas heretofore unseen by the light of day.

▶ Repeat for approximately five minutes.

▶ Wipe the tears from your eyes as she tweezes stray hairs and trims the "landing strip."

▶ Vow never to come again. Change your mind twelve hours later (at about 2 in the morning), and remind yourself to call tomorrow to book your next appointment.

∽ How To: Make Waxing or Lasering Only About <u>Half</u> As Painful As Childbirth

▶ Never go during your period. Your pain threshold is now at its lowest, so the ripping which normally hurts like hell will now hurt like &!*%! Wait until the week after your period, when the threshold is highest.

▶ Give yourself a short trim so that your hair is about a quarter to half an inch long. Nothing compounds the embarrassment like having Ilsa bent closely over your privates, examining everything to figure out how much to snip.

▶ An hour beforehand, pop an Advil or ibuprofen.

▶ Half an hour beforehand, spread LMX cream (which you can buy at most drugstores) all over the regions to be waxed or lasered. It'll numb the area and cut the pain in half, seriously.

▶ Bring your iPod. This might sound kind of silly, but trust me from experience—it works.

▶ Take a deep breath before each yank. (Hey, women in labor practice Lamaze for a reason!)

▶ Don't plan on going "completely bare" during your first ever wax—wait until another appointment.

▶ Avoid swimming in chlorinated water immediately before or after your wax, which can irritate the raw skin.

∾ Waxing Lingo

So, you think you know what all the terms mean, but do you really? Here's a rundown of all the terms and options. (Hey, makes it sound just like a car!)

Brazilian: Everything is removed (I mean, we're talking *everything . . . all the way back*), except for a thin line of hair on your pelvis.

Landing strip or The Playboy: The line of hair left during Brazilian bikini waxes. Commonly seen on *Playboy* Playmates.

The Natural: A conservative waxing job, removing only hair along the bikini border and "shaping" the remaining hairs.

Triangle: This is the typical shape you're familiar with that follows the curve of your thighs. More hair is removed than with "The Natural," but it's still a feminine look that shouldn't anger *too* many women's libbers.

Completely Bare (also known as the Full Monty or Full Bikini Wax): I think this one is pretty self-explanatory. For those of you still wrinkling your noses in confusion: the waxer tends to you until you're bare. *Completely* bare.

∾ What to Tip:

How do you gracefully and appropriately tip somebody who has just seen more of you than your boyfriend and gynecologist combined? Well, for starters, wait until you're fully clothed and out the door to tip. (Hey, you never know.) Even better, hand the tip to the receptionist in an envelope, if possible. Seeing the waxers in your street clothes . . . it's always a little jarring, no? Even though you might feel compelled to overtip out of embarrassment for making the poor aesthetician get *thisclose*, the standard 20% will do just fine here.

∽ What the Hell Is IPL?

If you're familiar with the menu on offer at waxing locations (or your dermatologist's office; see Chapter Five), you've probably heard about IPL. It stands for intense pulsed light and is a revolutionary way of removing freckles, broken capillaries, pigmentation . . . and most importantly, unwanted hair. I am, frankly, obsessed with it. It's non-ablative (a fancy way of saying it doesn't damage the surface of the skin), takes about ten or fifteen minutes for the bikini area, and after six treatments, your hair is gone for good. (All that's required are touch-up sessions every couple of years to keep the hair banished.) It's better for those with fair skin and dark hair, but advances are being made daily, and now most people can safely and effectively get rid of hair with IPL. If you decide to spring for it, you'll need at least six sessions (one a month, for six months), and it'll run you around $300 a pop. Take it from somebody's who's tried it, however—it is *so* worth it.

∽ Avoiding Ingrown Hairs

The unfortunate byproduct of a smooth, hairless body can be those nasty little bumps that crop up from inflamed skin and ingrown hairs. Luckily, I've never experienced more than a few ugly bumps here and there after shaving my bikini line haphazardly without cream, but a friend of mine has experienced painful, enlarged ingrowns her entire life. To treat them, look for products containing salicylic acid, such as Tend Skin, Completely Bare Bikini Bump Blaster, or Bliss Ingrown Hair Eliminating Peeling Pads. (You could also simply use anti-acne products with salicylic acid, such as Clearasil pads.)

∾ How To: Wax at Home

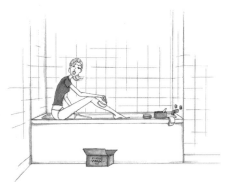

Okay, so unless you're a total sadist, waxing yourself isn't exactly *fun*, but it can be a hell of a lot less scary than you may think. Whether you're stripping hair from your bikini line, underarms, or legs, follow these simple rules to achieve that oh-so-coveted hairless Barbie look. And don't freak out if it hurts a bit and seems slightly complicated. With enough practice, you'll be putting the good ladies at your local salon to shame.

1. Trim it: Make sure the hair is about a centimeter or two long. It should be long enough to get a good grip to pull, but short enough so that it's easy to manage.
2. Get a kit: Many drugstore brands offer full kits including everything you need—from the wax and sticks to muslin cloth and even soothing ointment. Instead of conven-

tional wax, try using sugar or honey wax kits. These are thinner and easier to apply/remove!

3. Powder: Rub some baby powder or talc on the area you plan to wax. This will make the wax less likely to stick to your skin.

4. Do a quick test: Whether you're doing your bikini line or underarms, test a small section on your shin to gauge how the wax is working for you.

5. Cut the strips: Especially true for the bikini section! Hair might not always grow in the same direction, so be sure to cut smaller pieces to handle more manageable sections.

6. Apply and pull: Apply the wax with the wooden stick in the same direction as the hair growth. After smoothing on the waxing strip, be very quick in ripping off the cloth in the opposite direction of where you smoothed it. This will encourage slower regrowth.

7. Oil and soothe: To take off any persistent wax, just use baby oil. Aloe (also used for sunburns) will soothe any reddened skin post-waxing.

Chapter Ten Product Price Guide

$: less than $10
$$: between $10 and $24
$$$: between $25 and $49
$$$$: between $50 and $100
$$$$$: more than $100

LMX cream $, drugstores
Tend Skin, $$, *tendskin.com*
Completely Bare Bikini Bump Blaster, $$$, *completelybare.com*
Bliss Ingrown Hair Eliminating Peeling Pads, $$$,
    blissworld.com
Clearasil, $, drugstores

Eleven

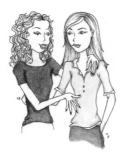

Manicure/Pedicure

If your nails don't look good, you don't look good

I have a friend. Let's call her May. May diligently goes to the nail salon once a week for a manicure, and once every two weeks for a pedicure. Like clockwork, she has her nails buffed, filed, soaked, and polished, always choosing tasteful colors like pale pink and nude. When she enters the salon, she is greeted like a rock star. I don't think May's nails have been without polish since 1993.

Then there's me. I love beauty, I love makeup, I love having pretty hands. I'm not a hippie or anything. (Not that there's anything wrong with hippies. But I am, in fact, the furthest thing possible from a hippie. Unless we're talking, like, a Kate Hudson-type hippie, because she's fabulous and I covet her chill Cali thing and her sexy, what?-I-just-have-great-hair-I-can't-help-it! thing. Good genes, that one. Anyhow.) Nails salons and all that girlie maintenance are great in theory—but manicures just take so *long*. And the polish chips *so often*. And

I can't even name the countless times I've left a pricey salon after a thorough (and thoroughly needed) manicure, only to smudge my polish three seconds after stepping on the street and then cursing the gods and wondering if I should go back in the salon to have them fix it, but then deciding that I simply cannot sit through twenty more minutes—or even twenty more seconds—of somebody tending to my nails like they're curing cancer. Can't somebody just invent a machine that I could stick my hands into for, say, five seconds, and then emerge perfectly groomed and polished? Anybody? If you could get on that, I'd be really grateful. I'm sure that millions of girls would buy it to avoid the duty of necessary pampering, too. Well, at least a few thousand. Or a few. Probably.

As for pedicures—forget it. I mean, I go there, like, once a year, tops.

I desperately wish I *were* one of those women who left the house with perfect nails, pink toes all clean and gleaming and heels smooth as a baby's bottom. My reality is usually much more horrifying, involving chipped polish, dry heels, and raggedy cuticles. (At least I can admit it. Acceptance is the first step toward recovery, no?) I tell myself it's because I'm busy. I'm busy, damn it! I am a very important person with very important things to do, such as . . . well, uh, writing and . . . um . . . reading . . . and, er, blogging—look, just trust me that I'm super busy. Manicures and pedicures are for socialites and Hollywood stars and trust-fund babies. The fact that I should be expected to have presentable nails when there are so many more important things to worry about in this world? It is akin to a crime! It is an outrage! We should all revolt!

Except . . . groomed nails really *do* look pretty. A fresh pedicure? Even better. On the rare occasions when I manage to

drag my lazy ass (No! Not lazy! Busy!) to the nail salon, I leave
a hand narcissist, unable to stop fluttering my fingers around
in the air admiringly and waving them in front of my face in
mirrors like some kind of deranged magician. (Or a recently
engaged chick.) I can't help it! They look so beautiful! My
hands are gorgeous! I should be a hand model! Why do I hate
manicures so much? I should do this once a week. I mean, it's
only an hour of my time, right? And then the polish chips . . .
and then I remember why.

Regardless of my personal biases, when it really matters
and when split-second impressions will be made (interviews,
parties, private dinners with Prince William—hey, you never
know), I make the mani/pedi effort. Nails are one of those
things that people see and instantly extrapolate to fifty other
aspects of your character. Short, clear nails? Conservative.
Long and red? Trashy. Raggedy cuticles? Messy. You could be
a Nobel-prize-winning scientist and speak seven languages,
but if you have a three-inch long snow-white-tipped French
manicure like some extra who's wandered off the set of *The
Sopranos*, you're simply not going to be taken as seriously. It's
not just the fact that your nails are groomed (although that's
half the battle)—it's *how* they're groomed as well. (Aww, man!
You mean we have to make twice the effort here?)

Luckily, the fact that taking care of your nails is so easy
and cheap means that almost any woman can afford to make
this a regular indulgence—whether at the local salon, or in the
privacy of your own home. Paradoxically, the more you do it,
the faster you can do it in, as well, since your nails will require
less upkeep. Of course, trying to fit in a quick jaunt to the nail
salon when you've got, say, a toddler (or even a needy boss or
a whiny husband) isn't always at the top of the priority list.

You're in the money, though, because when done properly, at-home manicures and the pricier, more time-consuming salon versions are barely distinguishable. If you've got ten minutes while Junior is napping or before your own bedtime, you have enough time to make your nails gorgeous—I promise.

⌒ At Home or at the Salon?

So, which are you? A salon-goer or an at-home gal? (Or, the elusive third category to which I belong: ambivalent.) Unless your personal manicurist is, say, nail-clipper-to-the-stars Deborah Lippmann, it *is* possible to replicate an at-home manicure or pedicure that's nearly as good as what you'll get at the salon. Of course, the advantage to doing your own nails is that it's much cheaper, plus you can fix them whenever the need arises, and you don't have to feel guilty that you're playing hooky from work during an extended "lunch break." Then again, half of the fun of getting your hands and feet done is, well, getting them *done*. It's like giving yourself a massage. What's the fun in that? Either way, whatever your preference, here are both scenarios, at home, and at the salon.

⌒ At Home

HOW TO: GIVE YOURSELF A PERFECT AT-HOME MANICURE

1. Soak nails in warm water for about three minutes to soften hands and cuticles.
2. Massage nails and hands with hand lotion.

3. Push cuticles back gently with an orange stick. You've heard it a million times, but avoid clipping your cuticles, since (even with your own tools) you could cause an infection.

4. File nails, taking care not to scrape the board back and forth across the top of the nail, which causes breakage; file nails in one direction only.

5. Clean nails thoroughly before polishing. If there are traces of lotion, your polish won't stick evenly. Use polish remover on a cotton ball to clean the surface.

6. Start with your thumb then work your way out to the pinky.

7. Apply basecoat to help polish go on more smoothly and last longer. (Many also include ingredients to help strengthen weak and brittle nails.)

8. Starting at the cuticle, polish on color. The trick is getting enough polish on the brush that it goes on smoothly, but not too much that the polish bubbles (wipe your brush along the inside of the bottle to remove excess polish). Wait about three minutes, so the polish can slightly dry, then follow with a second coat.

9. Finish with a topcoat to give a shiny finish. It will also help even out streaks and save time from having to repaint.

10. Take your time! It will take a minimum of half an hour for nails to dry properly. (You know how it goes: nails *seem* dry, you reach for your key, and bam!—nicks everywhere.)

▶ Round tips can make big hands or feet look delicate. Square tips don't break as easily as round, since filing down the sides tends to weaken the nail. Square tips and sheer, pinky polish is a modern, updated twist on the French manicure look.

▶ When done, soak your hands in ice cold water for a minute or two to help polish dry.

▶ If you accidentally apply polish outside your nail area onto the skin, don't freak out and smudge your other nails trying to clean it up. Polish doesn't stick to skin, so after your nails are dry, you'll be able to simply flake it off.

▶ I once read that nail polish can take up to four hours to completely dry. (Four!) Is this true? I don't know. What I do know is that I have, on many, many occasions, smudged my polish a full hour or two after a manicure. Treat nails delicately after polishing, just in case.

▶ Massage unpolished nails and cuticles weekly with olive oil to keep them moisturized and add a healthy shine.

▶ Put on a layer of clear polish or top coat every couple of days to help your manicure or pedicure last longer.

▶ Soak your nails in lemon juice to rid of yellow stains from polish.

▶ Prevent hangnails by keeping cuticles supple and moisturized. Never pull a hangnail—clip it with cuticle scissors instead.

HOW TO: PERFECT AT-HOME PEDICURE

▸ Soak feet in a basin of warm water filled with softening foot soak for 10 minutes.

▸ Remove old nail polish.

▸ Clip toenails and push back cuticles.

▸ Buff nails if necessary.

▸ Using a foot file, gently rub back and forth across heels, balls of feet, and the bottom of toes to remove dead skin. I know foot callus scrapers are tempting (so disgusting-yet-simultaneously-fun to peel off all the old skin!), but avoid, unless bleeding feet are your thing.

▸ Apply moisturizing foot lotion all over feet and ankles and nails.

Did You Know?

Fingernails grow nearly four times faster than toenails. Nails grow fastest on your middle finger, and slowest on your thumb.

▸ Remove any lotion from the nail bed with a cotton ball.

▸ Repeat steps 7–10 in manicure steps above, beginning with a basecoat, then following with two layers of polish and topcoat.

∽ The Best Nail Polish Brands

Not all nail polish is created equal. Sure, they all look interchangeable in the bottle, but things like consistency and chip factor can make a huge difference, especially when the color is a "Look at Me!" one that will show globs or chips immediately. Walk into any nail salon in the country, and you're pretty much guaranteed to find either Essie or OPI nail polish, both of which have a fantastic array of colors and go onto the nail smoothly. Other excellent brands: Deborah Lippmann, Rimmel, and Revlon.

∾ To Help Prevent Chips

You spent half an hour doing your nails. You waited for them to dry. You even put your keys and phone on the dining room table before getting started, so you wouldn't have to dig them out of your purse. And then, like a moron, you went and smudged everything. Fabulous. What to do? Well, there's no secret, magic solution that I know of (like that nail polish machine I was talking about earlier. Make it happen, Nail Polish People of America!), but there *are* things you can do to minimize your likelihood of chips and smudges. A layer of Seche Vite or Orly Sec N'Dry on top of nail polish will help set color, dry it faster, and make it last longer.

∾ At the Salon

Hey, big spender! Look at you! Somebody's got the time *and* money on her hands for a weekly or bi-monthly nail salon visit. Consider yourself very fortunate.

Here's everything you need to know.

It may seem kind of silly to bring a nail kit to your favorite salon and ask them to keep it there for you, but in fact, many salons have areas set aside for this very purpose. Bringing your own tools—drugstores and Sephora sell kits—is the best way to ensure that you don't get a nasty infection. Don't assume that just because the salon is chi-chi and expensive that it's necessarily any cleaner than your garden variety corner sa-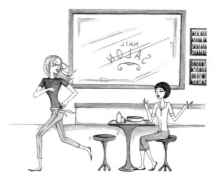lon; a few years back, a beauty editor went to one of New York's top nail salons and left with the not-so-glam present of a staph infection. Just as that oh-my-God-he's-so-sexy-he-should-be-a-model guy might be a hotbed of STD's, so could the place with the $60 manicure be a raging cesspool of bacteria. Makes you want to run straight to the salon, doesn't it?

This isn't to say that every salon is automatically dirty. If the tools are all prepackaged and sealed and the technician opens them in front of you, that's good. If you see technicians diligently cleaning the pedicure basins in between each customer, that's even better. And when the technician comes at you with a callus scraper or cuticle clipper, I hope the "Eee! Eee! Eee!" *Psycho* music flashes through your head and you politely, but firmly, stop her.

∾ The List: Best Nail Polish Colors

REDS

OPI I'm Not Really a Waitress: Sexy, vibrant, and the brightest shade of cherry red.

Revlon Red: A true, universally flattering red that—bonus— is chip-resistant.

NARS Dovima: With tomato-y undertones, this glamorous polish is better for olive and golden skin tones (or should we call them finger tones?).

PINKS

Essie Mademoiselle: A subtle, sophisticated flush of pink that's considered the most universally flattering shade (and is, as you've surely learned by my repeated mentions of it, my favorite nail polish in the world).

Chanel Le Vernis Nail Colour Boa: Flashy and attention-grabbing, like hot pink fruit punch, with blue undertones that look wonderful on both pale *and* tan skin.

Lippmann Collection Sarah Smile: A light, girly, sheer pink that was co-created with the patron saint of all that's cute and girly: Sarah Jessica Parker.

DARK

Chanel Black Satin: An instant classic that practically caused a national panic in the 90's, this still-popular polish is black as night.

Essie Licorice: Dark black, but with a sheen that makes it chic and not *too* goth.

OPI Lincoln Park After Dark: A bright, plummy, majestic purple, not for the faint of heart.

CHAPTER ELEVEN PRODUCT PRICE GUIDE

$: less than $10
$$: between $10 and $24
$$$: between $25 and $49
$$$$: between $50 and $100
$$$$$: more than $100

Essie Mademoiselle and Licorice, $, *essiecosmetics.com*
OPI I'm Not Really a Waitress and Lincoln Park After Dark, $, *opi.com*
Rimmel, $, drugstores
Revlon, $, drugstores
Seche Vite, $, drugstores
Orly Sec N'Dry, $, drugstores
Revlon Red, $, drugstores
NARS Dovima, $$, *narscosmetics.com*
Chanel Le Vernis Nail Colour in Boa and Black Satin, $$, *usa-chanel.com*
Lippmann Collection Sarah Smile, $$, *lippmanncollection.com*

Epilogue

The Importance of Beauty

• •

People often say that beauty is in the eye of the beholder, and I say that the most liberating thing about beauty is realizing that you are the beholder. This empowers us to find beauty in places where others have not dared to look, including inside ourselves.

Salma Hayek

• •

∾ My Personal Favorite Beauty Products

Now that you've read through *Beauty Confidential* (or just used it as a fly-swatter or decorative bathroom book— whatever), I hope you have a better sense both of what it's *really* like to be a beauty editor, and also of how you can act as your own personal beauty expert. Who needs a dermatologist or makeup artist or hairstylist or boyfriend (well, okay, maybe not the last one), when you can do it yourself?

You may have noticed that there are certain products I tend to be (either here in the book, or on my blog) more enthusiastic about than others. I confess: I play favorites. I'm an equal opportunity beauty gal, whoring out my beauty cabinet in the name of research with the best of them, but sometimes a product just grabs you and won't let go. (It's very rude, actually.) Here, my own personal best of the best.

Bare Escentuals: I can't stand foundation, but my red, acne-prone skin demands it. BE is the happy medium; it delivers whatever level of coverage you'd like, won't make you break out, and feels weightless. My number one product of all time.

OC 8: A godsend for oily skin, this zaps up shine all day long and works as a perfect makeup primer.

Narciso Rodriguez for Her: I've loved many perfumes in my life, but this sexy, musky beauty beats them all.

Chanel Coco Mademoiselle: Well, okay, if I had to pick *two* perfumes, this would be the runner-up. It's light, sensual, musky, and feminine at the same time, and somehow manages to be both sophisticated and youthful.

Lancôme Definicils Mascara: I love all of Lancôme's award-winning mascaras (the secret is in the special, patented brushes!), but none are better than lengthening Definicils, which makes lashes so long and defined that I sometimes even skip the lash curler. (This is huge, people.)

Shu Uemura Cleansing Oil: Gasp! Cleanse your oily skin with oil? You bet. It'll take off all your makeup, so there's no residue left on your face to clog pores.

Bumble and bumble Styling Spray: What's in this stuff? Magic? No other product will let you do so much with your hair; from straightening to sleekifying to thickening to curling. It's kind of like boot camp for your hair—guaranteed to whip it into shape.

IS Clinical Pro-Heal Serum: An antioxidant powerhouse, including up-and-coming olive leaf extract, this not only protects skin from sun damage and free radicals, but also helps keep your complexion smooth, even-toned and blemish-free. Truly something of a miracle in a bottle.

MD Skincare Alpha-Beta Peels: Clinical and decadent at the same time, these combination salicylic acid and glycolic acid peels help increase collagen production and cell turnover, which means fresher, clearer, firmer looking skin for you. Plus, they're just fun to use.

Essie polish in Mademoiselle: Sometimes, when I'm feeling bored, I cheat on Essie Mademoiselle. Then I look at my nails, and I miss her light, subtle pinkness. I always go back.

My (Living, Breathing) Style Obsessions

Kate Middleton: Sure, Kate may never be Queen, but she's still fascinating. (Now maybe even more so.) Not only is Kate gorgeous, in an accessible, non–Paris Hilton kind of way, but she's gradually evolving into an enviable style icon right before our eyes. She pulls off the horsey-country chic thing to a T, with her long, thick, shiny brown hair, tasteful makeup and understated-yet-appealing outfits. She's only going to become more stunning, and I can't wait to see where she goes from here.

Charlotte Casiraghi: Okay, I obviously have a soft spot for the young royals here, but who *wouldn't* be envious of a chick who's the granddaughter of Grace Kelly, the daughter of Princess Caroline, and looks like Angelina Jolie to boot? A star in the equestrian world, Charlotte is just as beautiful with her hair pulled into a messy bun and shoved under a riding cap as she is with her thick brows, pouty lips, and glossy chestnut hair done up to full splendor for a Monagasque or Parisian gala. Truly graceful, just like her grandmother.

Mandy Moore: Mandy Moore? Really? Yes, indeed. She's gorgeous on the outside, sure, but the fact that she's rarely photographed without a Julia Roberts–wattage smile makes her even prettier. Unlike many other young, wannabe-sexy Hollywood clones who think that beauty is a simple equation (no fat on body + long, blond hair extensions = cover of *US Weekly*), Mandy does it her own way, chopping off her flaxen tresses for a short, raven-colored bob, and flaunting a real, appealing, human body that doesn't look like it comes from Mars (take a look at her next to other actresses and singers—she completely dwarfs them, making them look like the anomalies that they actually are). Plus, she's just so damn cute (not to mention talented—see *Saved*, and tell me there's not a future Reese Witherspoon lurking in there) that no matter what kind of beauty look she's got going on, she's rocking it.

Kate Winslet: I'll admit it, I have a small girl crush on Kate Winslet. She's stunning, she's a world-class actor, she's down-to-earth, she's vulnerable, and she's terribly physically appealing. *Titanic* came out a decade ago (where does the time go?), and not only does Kate look as good as ever, but she actually looks better (and not in an overly plastic-y, I've had everything from my neck up "worked on" so much that I cannot blink or sneeze look, either.) Here's to a smart, delicious woman showing all the girls how it's *supposed* to be done.

Diane Lane: When I am in my forties, please let me be even a tenth as beautiful as Diane Lane is. Have you seen *Unfaithful?* The crinkles at the corner of her eyes, the laugh lines, the lived-in skin—I had no idea you could be so sexy and sensual at that age. Or, hell, even *more* sexy and sensual at that age than us young'uns. Cut me some slack here, I'm only in my twenties. I keep hearing that it only gets better . . . and Diane Lane definitely makes me believe it.

∾ So. Beauty, Huh?

In our increasingly cynical, political world, wanting to be pretty is not hip. It's politically incorrect to say that you feel anxious or annoyed or frustrated when tripped up by a bad hair day or mega zit that's impossible to cover up. I mean, how shallow are *you*? There are wars and genocide and natural disasters, and here you are moaning about your looks? Put it all into perspective, *please*.

Fine. Fair enough. It's not earth-shattering, disease-curing stuff. You having bad skin or tragic eyeliner (you know, when it smears up and hits the crease of your eyelid, and then you have a weird barcode-type line above your eye for hours without realizing it?) is not life or death. But who wants a life where all you do is focus on the serious stuff? What about art? Or music? Dance? Books? The theater? Necessities, none . . . but it's the stuff that makes life *exciting*.

Take away the makeup and the hair products and the joy of highlights and the rush of getting a makeover and walking into a room and having somebody not recognize you, and you might as well be a boy. (Well, minus the Playstation addiction and weird compulsion to burp and scratch your crotch.) Beauty is—and should be—a pleasure, not a chore. It's not about looking hot for men, or competing to look better than your friends; it's about doing it for yourself, because you take pride in your appearance, and you want to, and it looks good, damn it.

Every beauty editor has that moment when her job is coming crashing down on her and her (potentially diva) boss is yelling and the phone is ringing non-stop and she's just made an error involving mascara prices ($7.99, not $17.99—egads!) and assistants and editors are scuttling about in full-speed panic mode because the editor-in-chief has suddenly decided that she does not like the word "genius" anymore and wants to not only ban it from the magazine forever, but also take it out of the issue *right now*, which needs to happen in approximately the next fifteen seconds. The editor looks around at everybody freaking out, which in turn freaks *her* out, and she thinks, "This is ridiculous. It's not a hospital. It's just a stupid magazine. Everybody *calm down*."

Then, the next day, or maybe a week later, the new issue comes out and she flips through the pages and looks at what she's been working on for the past three months, then casually tosses it aside, only to be reminded about what she actually does later when a friend calls, or an acquaintance stops her in the street, or another editor mentions at an event: "I just read your article and I loved it! I never knew that tip about mascara . . ." Sure, it's kind of silly, but it makes her feel proud . . . just a little.

And then her mom sends an email, and at the end, she asks the editor to recommend a good product for thinning hair and sagging skin, since she's not feeling her best lately and she's going through a slump with the editor's father. When she has dinner with her best friend, the friend asks, "Do you think it's okay for me to switch to drugstore products? I'm too broke to afford anything from Bloomingdales or Sephora, but I don't want to ruin my skin." The cousin calls: "My best friend is *dying* to get into the industry. Would you mind having coffee with her next week to let her pick your brain? I'll tell her to bring her resume." She meets a friend of a friend at a wedding: "Oh, she told me about you! You're the beauty girl!"

And she's not a news reporter, or a detective, or a research scientist, or a politician. But it clicks—it's okay.

Everyone has something. Everyone finds a niche and

makes it their own. The editor? She's found her niche. She is the beauty girl . . . and in a small, but not insignificant way, it matters.

No, it's not life or death. It's just beauty. But it sure as hell makes life more fun.

Epilogue Product Price Guide

$: less than $10

$$: between $10 and $24

$$$: between $25 and $49

$$$$: between $50 and $100

$$$$$: more than $100

Bare Escentuals i.d. bareMinerals, $$$, *sephora.com*

OC 8, $$, *oc8.com*

Narciso Rodriguez for Her, $$$$, *saksfifthavenue.com*

Chanel Coco Mademoiselle, $$$$, *usa-chanel.com*

Lancôme Definicils, $$, *lancôme-usa.com*

Shu Uemura High-Performance Cleansing Oil Fresh, $$$$, *shuuemura-usa.com*

Bumble and bumble Styling Spray, $$, *bumbleandbumble.com* for locations

IS Clinical Pro-Heal Serum, $$$$, *isclinical.com*

MD Skincare Alpha-Beta Peel, $$$$, *mdskincare.com*

Essie Mademoiselle, $, *essiecosmetics.com*

∾ Note on the Products in This Book

Obviously, beauty products come and go, so it's always possible that these products could be discontinued at any point. All prices are approximate, and all locations were correct as of this writing, but, of course, that kind of stuff changes, too. However, I've tried to only include products that, for good reason, are considered "classics." Let's hope they stick around forever!

∽ INDEX OF PRODUCTS

Bobbi Brown Eyeshadow in Bone, $$, *bobbibrowncosmetics.com*

Bobbi Brown, $$ - $$$$, *bobbibrowncosmetics.com*

Bond No. 9 Chinatown, $$$$$, *saksfifthavenue.com*

Bond No. 9 West Side, $$$$$, *saksfifthavenue.com*

Britney Spears Fantasy, $$$, *sephora.com*

Bulgari Eau de Thé Verte, $$$$, *neimanmarcus.com*

Bulgari Omnia, $$$$, *neimanmarcus.com*

Bumble and bumble Does It All Styling Spray, $$, *bumbleandbumble.com* for locations

Bumble and bumble Hair Powder, $$, *bumbleandbumble.com* for locations

Bumble and bumble Styling Spray, $$, *bumbleandbumble.com* for locations

Bumble and bumble Styling Spray, $$, *bumbleandbumble.com* for locations

Bumble and bumble Thickening Spray, $$, *bumbleandbumble.com* for locations

Burt's Bees Beeswax Lip Balm, $, *burtsbees.com*

Burt's Bees Buttermilk Lotion, $, *burtsbees.com*

Calvin Klein Eternity Moment, $$$$

Carmex, $, drugstores

Cetaphil Face Wash, $, drugstores

Cetaphil Moisturizing Cream, $, drugstores

Chanel Allure Sensualle, $$$$, *usa-chanel.com*

Chanel Coco Mademoiselle, $$$$, *usa-chanel.com*

Chanel eye shadow, $$$, *usa-chanel.com*

Chanel Gardenia, $$$$, *usa-chanel.com*

Chanel Le Vernis Nail Colour in Boa and Black Satin,
usa-chanel.com

Chanel No. 19, $$$$, *usa-chanel.com*

Chanel Number 5, $$$$, *usa-chanel.com*

ChapStick, $, drugstores

Chi Ceramic Original Flat Iron, $$$$$, *farouk.com*
for locations

City Lips Lip Plumper, $$, *sephora.com*

Claremont Resort and Spa, 41 Tunnel Road, Berkeley,
California: 510-843-3000

Clarins Beauty Flash Balm, $$$, *clarins.com*

Claus Porto: $$, *lafcony.com*

Clean and Clear Oil-Free Dual Action Moisturizer, $,
drugstores

Clean and Clear Persagel, $, drugstores

Clean by D'Lish, $$$, *sephora.com*

Clearasil, $, drugstores

Clinique 3-Step System, $$$$, *clinique.com*

Clinique Acne Solutions Body Treatment Spray, $$,
clinique.com

Clinique Black Honey, $$, *clinique.com*

Clinique Happy, $$$, *clinique.com*

Clinique Make Up Brush Cleaner, $$, *clinque.com*

Clive Christian, $$$$$, *neimanmarcus.com, saksfifthavenue.com*

Coal tar, $, drugstores

Completely Bare Bikini Bump Blaster, $$$,
completelybare.com

Cortisone Cream, $, drugstores

Cowshed, $$$, *cowshedproducts.com*
Creed Fleurissimo, $$$$$, *neimanmarcus.com*
Creed Jasmal, $$$$$, *neimanmarcus.com*
Creed Spring Water, $$$$$, *neimanmarcus.com*
Crème de la Mer, $$$$$, *cremedelamer.com*
Crisco, $, grocery stores
DDF Fade Gel 4, $$$$, *sephora.com*
Dead Sea Salts, $, drugstores
Dermablend Smooth Concealer, $$, *dermablend.com*
Desert Essence Organic Jojoba Oil, $$, *desertessence.com*
DHC Deep Cleansing Oil, $$$, *dhccare.com*
Dior Addict, $$$$, *eluxury.com*
Dior DiorShow Mascara, $$, *eluxury.com*
Dior eye shadow, $$$, *eluxury.com*
Diptyque, $$$, *neimanmarcus.com*
Dolce and Gabbana Light Blue, $$$, *sephora.com*
Donna Karan Be Delicious, $$$, *donnakaran.com*
Donna Karan Black Cashmere, $$$$, *neimanmarcus.com*
Dove soap, $, drugstores
Dr Dennis Gross, 105 East 37th Street, New York, NY: 212-725-4555
Dr Hauschka: $$$, *drhauschka.com*
Dr Kenneth Beer, 1500 North Dixie Highway, West Palm Beach, FL, 561-655-9055
DuWop Lip Venom, $$, *sephora.com*
DuWop Reverse LipLiner, $$, *sephora.com*
Elidel: $$$, *elidel.com* for dermatologists
Elizabeth Arden Green Tea, $$, *elizabetharden.com*
Epsom Salts, $, drugstores

Essie Mademoiselle, $, *essiecosmetics.com*

Essie Licorice, $, *essiecosmetics.com*

Essie nail polish, $, *essiecosmetics.com*

Eucerin Aquaphor Healing Ointment, $, drugstores

Eucerin Redness Relief, $$, drugstores

Fake Bake, $$$, *fakebake.com*

Flawless by Danilo, $$$, *ultimatelooks.com*

Flaxseed or fishseed oil capsules, $$, health food stores

Floris, $$$$, *florislondon.com*

Fracas, $$$$$, *neimanmarcus.com*

Frederic Fekkai Glossing Cream, $$, *sephora.com*

Freeze 24/7, $$$$$, *freeze247.com*

Fresh Brown Sugar Body Polish, $$$$, *fresh.com*

Giorgio Armani Eyeshadow #12, $$$,
  giorgioarmanibeauty-usa.com for locations

Giorgio Armani Shine Gloss #4, $$,
  giorgioarmanibeauty-usa.com for locations

Givenchy Pi, $$$$, *givenchy.com* for locations

Glow by J.Lo, $$$, *shopjlo.com*

Gold Bond Ultimate Healing Skin Therapy Lotion, $,
  drugstores

Guerlain Mitsouko, $$$$$, *guerlain.com* for locations

Guerlain Shalimar Light, $$$$, *guerlain.com* for locations

Guerlain Shalimar, $$$$, *neimanmarcus.com*

**Hermès Eau d'Orange Verte Orange Givree Freshness
  Wake Up Gel,** $$, *usa.Hermès.com*

Hermès Eau d'Orange Verte, $$$$$, *usa-Hermès.com*

Hermès, $$$$$, *usa-Hermès.com*

Hydrocortisone cream, $, drugstores

Hylexin, $$$$, *sephora.com*

Infusium, $, drugstores

IS Clinical Active Serum, $$$$, *isclinical.com*

IS Clinical Pro-Heal Serum, $$$$, *isclinical.com*

Issey Miyake Eau d'Issey, $$$$, *neimanmarcus.com*

Jane Blushing Cheeks Powder Blush in Blushing Petal, $,
drugstores

Jason, $, *jason-natural.com*

**Jemma Kidd Makeup School Lasting Tint Semi-Permanent
Waterproof Mascara:** $$$, *neimanmarcus.com*

JF Lazartigue Stimulactine 21, $$$$, *jflazartigue.com*

Jo Malone Lime, Basil and Mandarin Shower Gel, $$$$,
jomalone.com

Jo Malone Red Roses, $$$$, *jomalone.com*

Jo Malone, $$$$, *jomalone.com*

John Frieda Secret Weapon, $, drugstores

Johnson and Johnson No More Tears Baby Shampoo, $,
drugstores

Johnson's Softlotion 24 Hour Moisture Body Lotion, $,
drugstores

Jurlique, $$$, *jurlique.com*

Kai, $$$, *abeautifullife.com*

Ken Paves salon, 409 North Robertson Boulevard,
Los Angeles, CA: 310-499-7122

Ken Paves, $$$$, *hairuwear.com*

Kerastase Olèo-Relax, $$$, *kerastase.com* for locations

Kerastase, $$$, *kerastase.com* for locations

Kiehl's Lip Balm # 1, $, *kiehls.com*

Kiehl's Original Musk Oil, $$, *kiehls.com*

Kinerase, $$$$$, *sephora.com*

Kiss Me Mascara, $$, *blincinc.com*

Klorane Extra Gentle Dry Shampoo Spray, $$, *metrobeauty.com*

L'Oreal brushes, $, drugstore

L'oreal Elnett hairspray: $$, *zitomer.com*

L'Oreal Nature's Therapy Mega Moisture Hair Treatment, $, drugstores

L'Oreal Paris True Match Concealer, $, drugstores

L'Oreal Professionnel Serie Expert, $$, *us.lorealprofessionnel.com* for locations

L'Oreal Voluminous, $, drugstores

La Roche Posay Anthelios L, $$$, *zitomer.com*

La Roche Posay Anthelios XL: $$$, *zitomer.com*

Lancôme eye shadow, $$$, *lancôme-usa.com*

Lancôme Definicils, $$, *lancôme-usa.com*

Lancôme Flash Bronzer Instant Colour Self-Tanning Leg Gel, $$$, *lancôme-usa.com*

Lancôme Trésor, $$$, *lancome-usa.com*

Laura Mercier Oil-Free Foundation Primer, $$$, *lauramercier.com*

Laura Mercier Secret Camouflage, $$$, *lauramercier.com*

Laura Mercier Secret Concealer, $$$, *lauramercier.com*

LipFusion XL, *sephora.com*

Lippmann Collection Sarah Smile, $$, *lippmanncollection.com*

LMX, $, drugstores

L'Oreal True Match Super-Blendable Concealer, $, drugstores

NARS Orgasm, $$, *narscosmetics.com*

Nature's Gate, $, *natures-gate.com*

Neem oil, $, organic health food stores

Neutrogena Norwegian Formula Hand Cream, $, drugstores

Neutrogena Oil-Free Acne Wash, $, drugstores

Neutrogena Oil-Free Moisture for Sensitive Skin, $,
drugstores

Nina Ricci L'Air du Temps, $$$$, *sephora.com*

Nioxin Recharging Complex, $$, *nioxin.com* for locations

OC8, $$, *oc8.com*

Olay In Shower Gel, $, drugstores

Olay Regenerist, $$, drugstores

Olay Total Effects Anti-Wrinkle/Anti-Blemish, $$, drugstores

OPI I'm Not Really a Waitress, $, *opi.com*

OPI Lincoln Park After Dark, $, *opi.com*

Oribe salon, 1627 Euclid Avenue, Miami Beach, FL:
305-538-8006

Origins, $$, *origins.com*

Orly Sec N'Dry, $, drugstores

Oscar Blandi Pronto Dry Shampoo, $$, *oscarblandi.com*

Osmotics Lipoduction Body Perfecting Complex, $$$$,
osmotics.com

Ouidad Climate Control Gel, $$, *ouidad.com*

Pantene, $, drugstores

Penhaligon, $$$$, *penhaligons.co.uk*

Philip B Rejuvenating Oil, $$$, *philipb.com*

Philosophy Save Me, $$$$, *sephora.com*

Phytodefrisant, $$$, *phyto-usa.com* for locations

Pssst! Dry Powder Spray, $$, drugstores
Purpose Redness Reducing Moisturizer SPF 30, $,
   drugstores
Ralph by Ralph Lauren, $$$$, *polo.com*
Ralph Lauren Romance, $$$, *polo.com*
Red Flower, $$$$, *redflower.com*
Revlon nail polish, $, drugstores
Revlon Red, $, drugstores
Rimmel, $, drugstores
ROC Age Diminishing Moisturizing Night Cream, $$,
   drugstores
ROC Retinol Correxion Intensive Anti-Wrinkle Care, $$,
   drugstores
Sally Hansen polish, $, drugstores
Salon Eliut Rivera, 762 Madison Avenue, New York, NY:
   212-472-3440
Santa Maria Novella: $$, *lafcony.com*
Sarah Jessica Parker Lovely, $$$,
   sarahjessicaparkerbeauty.com
Seche Vite, $, drugstores
Sephora brushes, $$ - $$$$$, *sephora.com*
Shiseido Body Creator Aromatic Firming Cream, $$$$,
   shiseido.com
Shiseido Eyelash Curler, $$, *shiseido.com*
Shu Uemura brushes, $$$, *shuuemura-usa.com*
Shu Uemura Eyelash Curler, $$, *shuuemura-usa.com*
Shu Uemura High-Performance Cleansing Oil Fresh, $$$$,
   shuuemura-usa.com
Slatkin and Co, $$$, *neimanmarcus.com*

Smashbox I Prime Under Eye Primer and Concealer, *sephora.com*

Smashbox Photo Finish Primer, $$$, *sephora.com*

Smashbox, $$ - $$$$, *smashbox.com*

Solano Sapphire Flat Iron, $$$$, *folica.com*

Stella McCartney Stella, $$$$, *neimanmarcus.com*

Stila Kajal eyeliner, $$, *stila.com*

Stila Lip Pot in Mure, $$, *stila.com*

T3 Tourmaline Evolution Hair Dryer, $$$$$, *nordstrom.com*

T3 Tourmaline Featherweight Professional Ionic Hair Dryer, $$$$$, *nordstrom.com*

Tazorac, $$$, *tazorac.com* for dermatologists

Tend Skin, $$, *tendskin.com*

Terax Crema, $$, *sephora.com*

Terax Original Crema, $$, *sephora.com*

Terax Original Lotion Life Drops, $$, *sephora.com*

The Body Shop, $$, *thebodyshop.com*

Trish McEvoy Even Skin Face Primer, $$, *trishmcevoy.com*

Vera Wang, $$$, *neimanmarcus.com*

Victoria Secret Very Sexy for Her, $$$, *victoriasecretbeauty.com*

Warren-Tricomi salon, 16 West 57th Street, New York, NY: 212-262-8899

Weleda Skin Food, $$, *usa.weleda.com*

YSL Nu, $$$$, *nordstrom.com*

YSL Touche Eclat Radiant Touch, $$$, *nordstrom.com*

Yves Saint Laurent Opium, $$$$, *neimanmarcus.com*

Yves Saint Laurent Touche Éclat Radiant Touch, $$$, *nordstrom.com*

Dubbed "the poster girl for the blogger generation" by the *New York Post*, NADINE HAOBSH was born in New York City in 1980. After twenty-two years of obsessively staring at her hair in the mirror (and following internships at CNN, *InStyle*, *Harper's Bazaar*, and *FHM*), she discovered that it was indeed possible to make a career out of narcissism and became a beauty editor. Stints at *Lucky* magazine and *Ladies' Home Journal* seemed promising until Nadine began a blog under the pseudonym "Jolie in NYC," where she dispensed beauty advice and celebrity gossip. Mayhem ensued, her identity was revealed, the beauty industry went into an uproar, and an offer at *Seventeen* magazine was rescinded. (It was a busy day.) Since being outed, internationally chronicled, and thrust into the spotlight as a beauty expert, Nadine blogs twice daily for *Jane* magazine online, works as a beauty and media consultant, and maintains the blog "Jolie in NYC," which has received over three million hits. She has a passion for traveling and learning new languages, and currently divides her time between Palm Beach, New York City, and London. Her second book, a novel entitled *The Beauty Expert*, will be published by HarperCollins in 2008.